THE
PASTORAL
CAREGIVER'S
CASEBOOK

JOHN J. GLEASON, Editor

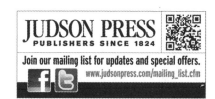

JUDSON PRESS
PUBLISHERS SINCE 1824

Join our mailing list for updates and special offers.
www.judsonpress.com/mailing_list.cfm

The Pastoral Caregiver's Casebook, Volume 2: Ministry in Crises
© 2015 by Judson Press, Valley Forge, PA 19482-0851
All rights reserved.

Judson Press has made every effort to trace the ownership of all quotes. In the event of a question arising from the use of a quote, we regret any error made and will be pleased to make the necessary correction in future printings and editions of this book.

Bible quotations in this book are quoted from NRSV the New Revised Standard Version Bible, copyright © 1989, Division of Christian Education of the National Council of the Churches of Christ in the United States of America. Used by permission. All rights reserved.

Interior design by Beth Oberholtzer.
Cover design by Danny Ellison.

Library of Congress Cataloging-in-Publication Data
The pastoral caregiver's casebook / John J. Gleason, editor.
    volumes cm
    Includes index.
    Contents: volume 1. Ministry in relationships—volume 2. Ministry in crises—volume 3. Ministry in health—volume 4. Ministry in specialized settings.
    ISBN 978-0-8170-1759-0 (volume 1 : paperback : alk. paper)—ISBN 978-0-8170-1760-6 (volume 2 : paperback : alk. paper)—ISBN 978-0-8170-1761-3 (volume 3 : paperback : alk. paper)—ISBN 978-0-8170-1762-0 (volume 4 : paperback : alk. paper) 1. Pastoral counseling—Case studies. 2. Pastoral care—Case studies. 3. Hospital patients—Pastoral counseling of—Case studies. 4. Caring—Religious aspects—Christianity—Case studies. I. Gleason, John J., 1934– editor.
    BV4012.2.P284 2015
    259—dc23

                         2014025834

Printed in the U.S.A.
First printing, 2015.

Contents

SECTION TWO
Ministry in Psycho-Spiritual Crises

Contents

Preface

Welcome to *The Pastoral Caregiver's Casebook*. May this collection of actual pastoral care case situations—each with critique and tentative effectiveness rating, and many with pertinent literature references—serve you well in your efforts to render the most effective spiritual care. (Note: The terms *pastoral care* and *spiritual care* are used interchangeably in this collection.)

The collection, originally titled the "Spiritual Care Initiative for Professional Excellence (SCIPE) Knowledge Base of Spiritual Care Samples," was edited by John J. Gleason, a retired Association for Clinical Pastoral Education Inc. supervisor and board-certified chaplain of the Association of Professional Chaplains. John Ehman, coordinator of the ACPE Research Network, created the initial categories, and Henry Heffernan, SJ, a staff chaplain at the National Institute of Health's Clinical Center, edited the first 25 samples. The material, submitted by chaplains and other pastoral caregivers from across the nation, is completely anonymous. Pastoral care case writers approved all edits before their entry into the collection.

Volume 2, *Ministry in Crises*, is divided into two major sections: Ministry in Physical Crises and Ministry in Psycho-Spiritual Crises. Other volumes in the series cover ministry in relationships (Volume 1), in different healthcare contexts (Volume 3), and in specialized settings (Volume 4). Each case is titled with a phrase that identifies the central issue in that scenario, as identified by the practitioner. Use the table of contents or index to find the case most like the one in which you are currently engaged, and seek a second opinion for your current ministry situation by reviewing the relevant material. Then make use of the insights and ideas that you deem worthy as you proceed with your own ministry.

Achievement of effective, evidence-based outcomes is becoming increasingly important among all professional caregiving disciplines. This is especially difficult in pastoral care, given the highly subjective nature of the ministry. Nonetheless, as a very early step in this direction, each case report includes a simple content analysis in which words and phrases that suggest effectiveness have been italicized to highlight how the recipient of care responded—for example, with thanks, affirmation, or expressions of emotional clarity or spiritual illumination.

Not every contributor included details that could be highlighted this way, but readers are encouraged to note such words and behaviors in their own caregiving encounters. Patient and parishioner responses can not only offer personal encouragement and affirmation to the spiritual caregiver, but those responses can also become the basis for measuring effectiveness in professional reporting and ministry assessment. (For instance, the editor used contributor reporting of such responses as a basis for excluding several cases from this volume, where insufficient information was provided or ineffective care was indicated.)

Use the collection for the training of seminarians and clinical pastoral education students. Experienced pastoral caregivers might follow this model in attempting self-supervision (for instance, by writing up your own cases for reflection and quality improvement). And the cases described here may also educate and enlighten the laity, healthcare administrators, and the general public about the nature and depth of spiritual care.

Ministry in Physical Crises

Among pastoral and spiritual caregivers, the term *crisis* is generally understood to be the experience of distress caused by a disruption in the balancing mechanisms that govern our daily lives. In this section, this disruption is caused by the anticipation or reality that this delicate balance cannot be maintained, primarily for physical reasons. The spectrum of these physical reasons ranges from a person's own minor illness or injury all the way to the removal of a loved one from a person's life, for whatever reason.

In your ministry to persons in such physical crises, may you find among these 32 cases and their reported learnings significant insights that drive you toward increased quality in your service as a conduit for divine healing power in people's lives.

Aging Issues

Description of the client's circumstances and the spiritual care offered:

The 65-year-old female patient had been admitted to the hospital for high blood pressure and chest pain. She felt depressed, was not taking her medications, and wished to die. A major stated concern was her lack of a boyfriend or a husband. She felt strongly that the reason for this lack was the fact that she was getting old and did not look beautiful. This was her state of mind when the chaplain entered.

At the chaplain's introduction of herself, the patient indicated that she was having a rough day. In addition to sharing the above information about herself, the patient also expressed concern about her life thus far. Her parents had not helped her much when she was growing up, and this had contributed to her depression. She also had unresolved issues from living with four boyfriends in past relationships that did not work out in her favor. These were the many concerns that kept her from taking her medication and made her wish to die. If she were to live, she wanted to start going out to clubs and movies to get what she wanted: a boyfriend or a husband.

The chaplain listened to her story with compassion and empathy, assuring the woman that she was indeed beautiful and that she had realistic dreams. The chaplain further urged her to start taking her medications. At that point, the patient *stated that the chaplain had helped her greatly.* Her *brightened affect* seemed to confirm her words. The visit was concluded with a knock at the door as the medical staff entered.

Description of what the practitioner, upon reflection, considers most appropriate:

The chaplain's upbeat approach seemed to have a very positive, if not miraculous, impact. However, optimism about the dramatic effect of this visit might well be tempered with a reminder that, realistically, one visit seldom turns a life around completely.

It would be important for the chaplain to continue visits during the course of the patient's hospitalization and for the chaplain to offer input into her release planning. Such planning could include connection with a congregation in the patient's community. This type of connection could help consolidate the gains made in the hospital by providing ongoing support and opportunities to form faith-based friendships.

Background information that the practitioner considers useful:

Erik H. Erikson, *Childhood and Society.* New York: Norton, 1963. Chapter 7.

Felicity B. Kelcourse, *Human Development and Faith.* St. Louis: Chalice, 2004. Chapter 1.

George A. Maloney, *Alone with the Alone.* Notre Dame, IN: Ave Maria, 1982. 122.

Glendon L. Moriarty and Louis Hoffman, eds., *The God Image: Self, Depression, and Christian Thought.* New York: Haworth, 2008. Chapter 3.

Anxiety about Resident's Own Funeral Plans

Description of the client's circumstances and the spiritual care offered:

The chaplain received a referral from a nurse who said that an elderly female resident, just transferred into the facility's long-term care unit, wished to see him. When the chaplain arrived at the room, the resident was gracious and readily engaged in small talk. The chaplain responded in kind, and persuaded by his encouraging and easygoing manner, the resident *began to share her story in more depth.* She told of her early experiences in the church and then described the current state of her congregation.

With sufficient rapport established, she *anxiously asked* the chaplain if he would be the one to conduct her funeral, saying that her greatest fear was that someone who didn't even know her would be the one to officiate. The chaplain readily agreed to her request, emphasizing that he would be honored to have that privilege.

Description of what the practitioner, upon reflection,
considers most appropriate:

Generally, the chaplain thought the conversation went well but felt that he may have been a little too "breezy" and conversational, especially at the point when she anxiously made her request.

Although he did tell the resident how honored he was by her request, in retrospect he realized that he sometimes failed to appreciate the anxiety elderly people feel about their funeral and burial plans.

Appropriate Religious Support at an Imminent Death

Description of the client's circumstances
and the spiritual care offered:

The new chaplain was called to the ICU to support the family of a dying patient. He was informed that death was imminent. He saw the husband and brother at the bedside of a young woman in her late thirties. Both men were somewhat distressed as they anticipated the chaplain's arrival. He approached and identified himself. They *requested prayer*. As the chaplain was all "prayed up" and ready, he began to pray. At the end of his prayer, they *began to chant*.

In his haste to be supportive, the chaplain had failed to ask their religious background and had gone right to his own Christian prayer mode. He apologized as soon as the chanting was over. They said it was not a problem, their being affiliated with an Eastern/Western religious amalgam. Their guru and the Christian Lord, Jesus Christ, were both worshiped.

When the chaplain apologized to the patient, she also said it was not a problem. In fact, the group *embraced the chaplain*, treating him with honor in each visit. The patient lived another five days. Her room saw 15 to 25 people journey with her until her death, chanting, praying, singing, and supporting.

Description of what the practitioner, upon reflection, considers most appropriate:

In retrospect the chaplain would have asked the family's religious affiliation at the outset of his initial visit. He also would not have been so quick to pray when asked, or use his "typical Christian lingo" in prayer. Lastly, he would have asked what the patient and family would have liked to include in the prayer.

Care for a Patient and Family of Faith at the Moment of Death

Description of the client's circumstances and the spiritual care offered:

The chaplain was called to assist a family during the removal of medical life-support for a male patient with bleeding in the brain. In a meeting with the chaplain before the patient entered the ICU, the family—wife, children, mother, sisters, and brothers—*requested prayer and singing* to let the patient go. They chose the hymn "Amazing Grace."

At the bedside, the chaplain spoke to the patient about what she and the family were going to do and why. He was unresponsive. They sang the hymn and the chaplain prayed. In tears, family members told the patient it was okay to go, and that they would see him in heaven someday.

After the breathing tube was removed, the nurse placed the patient's arms outside the covers so the family could touch and hold his hands. At that point, the patient slightly "shrugged" his shoulders—his first movement and response of any kind in three days. He never took another breath, but as prayers continued and the chaplain recited Psalm 23, the patient raised his arms as if to hug someone or something, and then pulled his hands together and drew them up under his chin. He died with such a look of peace on his face that all in the room were deeply moved.

Description of what the practitioner, upon reflection, considers most appropriate:

The experience had been such a blessing and affirmation of movement from this life toward the hoped-for life that the chaplain, in retrospect, could not imagine doing anything differently. The family had been so comforted by the patient's actions (and the chaplain's ministrations) that the faith of all present had been profoundly affirmed.

Background information that the practitioner considers useful:

1 Corinthians 15:35-58.

Don Piper with Cecil Murphey. *Ninety Minutes in Heaven*. Grand Rapids: Revell, 2004.

Caretaker for Dying Mother Wanting "Magic Words"

Description of the client's circumstances and the spiritual care offered:

An RN phoned the chaplain, who had just begun his evening on-call shift, to ask if he might come to the surgical recovery area to talk about her mother. (They had spoken previously about her dying mother.) Upon entering the surgical recovery area, the nurse greeted the chaplain with a smile. He asked her how she was doing. The RN explained that she needed some words from him about how to handle the situation with her mother, who was in a nursing home, not eating, and threatening to leave by calling 911 on her cell phone. The RN didn't know how to tell her mother that she was dying. The nurse repeated, "I needed some words from you about how to handle this situation."

The chaplain responded with empathic and affirming comments. The RN again expressed her hope that he had some words to help, this time calling them "magic words" for her. The conversation was punctuated by several interruptions to check on her patient and once to introduce a second nurse.

The crux came with her remark, "So, no magic words?" The chaplain replied, "I'm afraid not. I care, though. Do you have anyone to help you with this? Does your mom have a pastor?" The RN then *shared the story* of her mother's church "falling apart," the resulting isolation, and the RN's pain at her mother's own "falling apart." After another interruption to check on her patient, she asked again, "So, you have no guidance for me?" The chaplain responded, "I can't tell you what to say. I will tell you that I had to break this kind of news to my own mother." After sharing some details, he acknowledged, "That was my scenario. It's not yours . . . but whatever you do, do it with all of the tenderness in your heart." The conversation ended with details about her mother's name and mutual well-wishes.

Description of what the practitioner, upon reflection, considers most appropriate:

The chaplain clearly provided a caring, empathic, and appropriately self-revealing ministry. Regarding the crux of the conversation, he later observed, "I'm truly not sure if I was escaping the feelings of the moment (by asking about other possible helpers)." A question such as "What's that like for you?" or "How does that feel?" might have led to catharsis. On the other hand, such catharsis could have distracted her from her important post-op duties. It would have been helpful to set up a time and place where both could share and pray without distraction.

The chaplain indicated that he planned to follow up with her.

Background information that the practitioner considers useful:

Ernest Kurtz and Katherine Ketcham, *The Spirituality of Imperfection: Storytelling and the Search for Meaning.* New York: Bantam, 1992. 82–97.

Chaplain with Terminally Ill Husband

Description of the client's circumstances
and the spiritual care offered:

The chaplain's husband suffered with non-Hodgkin's lung lymphoma, fighting for recovery over a number of years but ultimately succumbing to the disease. To another chaplain she *described her personal effort* and that of the family as quite extensive through personal attention, the treatment, and care at the end of the illness. That effort included being "faithful to God if we did not understand why . . . this situation happened."

Description of what the practitioner, upon reflection,
considers most appropriate:

In retrospect the chaplain reported her failure as being overly confident in the efforts of the doctor and the family, because she could not believe her husband would really die. All that time, the chaplain thought he would be in recovery. Her husband shared that confidence. He told his wife that he did not like to talk about the end, and she tried to respect his feelings.

She added that it is still hard for her to accept that he is not with her, but she expressed her strong belief that she will see him again in Jesus' second coming. The chaplain further stated that illnesses are experiences of faith, and that the battle with illness is a victory in Jesus Christ. Her experience affirmed just how important it is to be a godly presence with patients and their families.

Community Clergy Initial Visit to a Dying Nursing Home Resident

Description of the client's circumstances
and the spiritual care offered:

A Lutheran community clergy was called to visit a dying 98-year-old nursing home resident. Knowing only that the resident was a religious person who attended services at the home—but had no known church or pastor—had two sons living away, and had a nephew nearby, after preparatory prayer the clergy arrived at the resident's bedside. Although mute, the resident was *somewhat responsive* to the clergy's ministrations, mostly via subtle eye movements. These ministrations included prayer, readings from Scripture and "Commendation for Dying" in her *Occasional Services Book*, singing, and gentle words of faith assurance.

During the visit, a nurse looked in briefly, and a bit later the nephew arrived. In conversation with the clergy, the nephew sketched his aunt's life of hard work, caring for others, living independently until a fall at age 95, and attendance at a particular church though she was not a member. The nephew *asked the clergy* if she could conduct his aunt's funeral. She agreed, and phone numbers were exchanged. Before parting, the clergy offered a prayer at the bedside in which she prayed for the family members as well as for the resident, and then agreed to make follow-up visits. She departed amid *expressions of appreciation* from the nephew and from the staff.

Description of what the practitioner, upon reflection,
considers most appropriate:

In retrospect the clergy thought that it might have helped had she known the resident previously. That might have allowed her to talk with the resident before she could no longer speak, because in that case the clergy could have brought up the subject of death and dying and then been able to hear what the resident's thoughts and wishes were.

The clergy also thought she might have asked more questions of the nurse who came into the room during her visit. Further, she could have asked the nephew if he knew what the resident's wishes were. Perhaps she could have talked about *last things* in the first visit instead of waiting until later visits.

One caution from the clergy: "Don't say anything within the hearing of the silent one that might more appropriately be said outside the room."

Background information that the practitioner considers useful:

Elisabeth Kübler-Ross, *On Death and Dying*. London: Macmillan, 1969.

Lutheran Book of Worship: Occasional Services. Minneapolis: Augsburg Fortress, 1990.

Confusion at a Deathbed Scene

Description of the client's circumstances and the spiritual care offered:

While on rounds, the night chaplain was asked by a nurse to visit the families of two critically ill patients. A short time later he arrived at the room of the second critically ill patient, and found the tearful and exhausted-looking spouse of the nonresponsive male patient who was in his late seventies. The wife had a heavy southern accent, and for most of the conversation the chaplain could not understand what she was saying. To further complicate matters, the chaplain noticed that the patient seemed to not be breathing, and he was unsure whether the spouse knew, since he had not been paged for the death according to protocol.

After 15 minutes of the chaplain's trying to understand the situation and the spouse, the wife suddenly spoke clearly, saying, "The verse that comes to mind is, 'He has fought the fight and has finished the race. Now is prepared for me a crown of righteousness.'" At least one question had been answered: she knew her husband was dead. The family began to gather in the room. After introductions the chaplain excused himself to get family members refreshments and to find out whether the death page had indeed been made. The nurse said that she had made the request, and abruptly turned away to speak with another nurse.

The chaplain returned to the room with the refreshments and listened as the family *expressed disappointment* that their own pastor had not come, as well as gratitude that the patient was no longer in pain. They *asked for prayer* and the chaplain met their request, with *amens* coming from various family members throughout the prayer.

Description of what the practitioner, upon reflection, considers most appropriate:

Despite a number of confusing and obstructive factors—inability to understand the spouse, breach of protocol, staff indifference, blurring of the chaplain's focus—the chaplain had been able to render significant spiritual care in a difficult situation, as attested to by the amens of affirmation in his prayer. The chaplain had sat quietly with the spouse, not understanding her but believing he was showing respect for her, while unclear about whether the patient was dead or alive and worried about what to do. At his first opportunity, he tried, unsuccessfully, to learn whether the death notification protocol had been followed correctly.

In retrospect the chaplain felt that his fear of asking for clarity from the spouse had limited his ability to help her. For example, he could have asked, "I am sorry. I speak in a different accent and I am not sure if I hear you correctly. What you are saying is important to me. Could you speak more slowly?" One bit of pressure could have been relieved if the chaplain had inwardly determined to pursue the protocol issue at a later time.

Background information that the practitioner considers useful:

Richard Dana, Lewis Bernstein, and Rosalyn S. Bernstein, *Interviewing: A Guide for Health Professionals.* Appleton-Century Crofts, 1985. 107–113.

Critically Ill ICU Patient's Daughter

Description of the client's circumstances
and the spiritual care offered:

An ICU patient's daughter requested a chaplain. She was tearful and anxious, not knowing how to respond when her very ill mother kept saying that she was tired and "didn't want to do this anymore." The daughter *noted her further anguish* that the doctor was not forthcoming with her mother's prognosis, and that she had questions about whether to consult hospice and palliative care. The chaplain encouraged the daughter to ask the doctor for clarity, empowering her as her mother's healthcare advocate.

Her father had been no help, saying only, "He's the doctor." Since the daughter and the chaplain were about the same age, the chaplain shared some similar experiences she had had with her own parents, and the self-revelation proved to be helpful in normalizing the father's behavior.

Although her mother was Christian Scientist and her father was Jewish, the daughter had no formal religious ties. However, she *fondly recalled a childhood memory* of a table at the front of her mother's church that had "God Is Love" inscribed on it. The daughter understood herself to be expressing her love and gratitude for her mother through that memory. The chaplain reflected that the love shared between her and her mother was a further reflection of God's love. An offer of prayer was declined. After the chaplain blessed the daughter and left, she informed the unit social worker of some of the daughter's concerns and questions.

Description of what the practitioner, upon reflection,
considers most appropriate:

Ideally, the chaplain would have done less probing for data, would have encouraged the daughter to name her feelings, and would have been more patient as the daughter shared more details about her mother. In her consultation with the floor social worker, the chaplain would have been more specific about the daughter's openness to hospice and palliative care.

Background information that the practitioner considers useful:

Mary Caswell Walsh, *Hidden Springs of Hope*, 1st ed. Notre Dame, IN: Ave Maria, 2001.

Developmental Crisis of Aging

Description of the client's circumstances
and the spiritual care offered:

A chaplain visited an 89-year-old woman in the hospital for treatment of pneumonia one day prior to her scheduled transfer to a rehabilitation facility. (She was experiencing difficulty walking after knee replacement surgery.) Always a take-charge, highly capable person, the patient was facing the prospect of increasing frailty. In the midst of her practical concerns, such as where she would live and how much assistive care she would need, she wanted to "get right with God" but felt great guilt for having been an indifferent practitioner of her Roman Catholic faith. She had worked out an idiosyncratic relationship with God that had served her well, but now she was worried because she had not strictly followed all of her church's rules, asking, "Am I strange?" She feared that her health problems were some sort of punishment from God for her less-than-orthodox spirituality.

After exploring her background and her faith, the chaplain offered his sense that she had indeed maintained a close and fruitful relationship with God, and suggested that under those circumstances God was unlikely to punish her. The chaplain invited her to revisit the prayer practices that had served her so well throughout her life. She was *happy to have the chaplain formulate a joint prayer*, but she was not forthcoming with prayer of her own. The patient seemed more frightened about having to cede control over her life than of being rejected by God. To initiate prayer seemed pointless to her.

Description of what the practitioner, upon reflection,
considers most appropriate:

The chaplain could have helped her to further revisit and reclaim
the meaningful aspects of her life. Blessing her efforts to be whole,
irrespective of her particular spiritual expression, and helping her
to integrate her prayer life with her practical concerns would have
enabled her to better understand the value that she, as a person of
integrity, had brought to the world.

Background information that the practitioner considers useful:

Jean Illsley Clarke and Connie Dawson, *Growing Up Again: Parenting
    Ourselves, Parenting Our Children*, 2nd ed. Center City, MI: Hazelden,
    1998.
Erik H. Erikson, *Identity and the Life Cycle*. New York: Norton, 1980.
James N. Lapsley, "Pastoral Care and the Counseling of the Aging," *Clinical
    Handbook of Pastoral Counseling*, Robert J. Wicks, Richard D. Parsons,
    and Donald E. Capps, eds. Mahwah, NJ: Paulist Press, 1985. 245–266.
Pamela Levin, "The Cycle of Development," *Journal of Transactional
    Analysis* 12, 1982. 136–137.

Displaced Grieving and Denial at a Family Matriarch's Death

Description of the client's circumstances
and the spiritual care offered:

The patient, a 76-year-old mother and grandmother, died early
on a Sunday morning. Her 45-year-old mildly brain-damaged
son *asked the chaplain for help* in talking to his nine-year-old
daughter about death. She was not present yet. When the man's
older brother arrived with his wife, they also were more focused
on their niece's response than on talking about their own feelings.
When the man's ex-wife arrived with the nine-year-old, her first
words were to tell her daughter to kiss her grandmother. The
chaplain took the nine-year-old and her father to a room across
the hall so the father could tell her about her grandmother's

death. Upon their return, all of the family members continued to focus on the little girl.

Description of what the practitioner, upon reflection, considers most appropriate:

Ideally, when the adults kept shifting the conversation back to the nine-year-old and her thoughts, the chaplain could have asked them—and especially the patient's two adult sons—about their own feelings about the patient's death. Because the young girl was supported by her mother, the chaplain could have exercised more pastoral authority in conversation with the sons.

Background information that the practitioner considers useful:

Erin Linn, *150 Facts about Grieving Children*. Incline Village, NV: Publisher's Mark, 1990.

Elderly Couple, Both Facing Terminal Illness

Description of the client's circumstances and the spiritual care offered:

A married couple in their seventies, long-time members of a congregation, discovered within a month that both had stage IV cancers. These physically active and vibrant senior adults now experienced the grief of realizing that their lives were forever changed. The pastor's first visit after they received the news was the most difficult, particularly as he grasped for words of comfort. The pastor spent most of the time *listening to their fears, recognizing their anger,* and *crying with them.*

Over time the visits became easier as they prayed together over specific issues: course of treatment, family responses, needs, and hopes. One of the most effective times was sitting with each of them as they thought out the important things they wanted to do before they died. With their pastor's help, the couple made sure these things occurred. For example, a rocker was placed in the aisle at church so they could continue to worship side by side.

In this process they became a faithful witness to the rest of the congregation.

At each death scene, the pastor led singing of hymns. The pastor's most powerful memory on each occasion was watching their lips move to the hymns.

Description of what the practitioner, upon reflection, considers most appropriate:

In retrospect the pastor felt that the experience had changed her as much as it had changed the husband and wife themselves: "Together we experienced God's grace."

If given the chance, the pastor "would have spent more time listening and just being with them." Instead, the demands of her schedule "always seemed to invade."

Background information that the practitioner considers useful:

L. Aden, "Comfort/Sustaining," *Dictionary of Pastoral Care and Counseling.* Nashville: Abingdon, 1990. 193–195.

End-of-Life Reflection Brought On by Recent Losses

Description of the client's circumstances and the spiritual care offered:

A male resident, between 60 and 70 years old, of a long-term care facility was visited on rounds by the chaplain, who had established an extensive pastoral relationship with the man over the course of several months. On this occasion, the ensuing pastoral encounter began with the resident dialoguing about his end-of-life concerns ("I'm thinking . . . about dying well"), which were rooted in the resident's recent loss of friends.

The chaplain offered sympathy and then asked if the resident wanted control over his own death. The resident stated that he had been treated "like a child" and was unable to be independent in his family of origin. The chaplain then asked, "So you would like your death to be different from your life. Is that fair [to say]?" This question *generated significant reflection* for the resident, such that he grew silent for a time. He did say late in the visit that he felt the presence of community in the dying process, as his fellow residents spoke openly about dying as well. The visit ended with the resident extending gratitude toward the chaplain by saying, "*Thank you* for being a friend." The chaplain responded, "Thank you for sharing with me, and it means a lot that you would consider me a friend. If you need me before (my next regular visit), just let a nurse know to page a chaplain."

Description of what the practitioner, upon reflection, considers most appropriate:

The visit and the relationship were validated by the resident's strongly affirming closing statement. At the same time, upon reflection the chaplain felt that he could have provided more effective pastoral care by using words and reflections that the resident provided rather than those the chaplain had created.

Additionally, the chaplain could have made a more appropriate affirmation of friendship within the clinical context for this resident. Rather than stating, "It means a lot that you would consider me a friend," a more appropriate affirmation might have been, "It is a privilege to be your friend."

Family Request that an Unresponsive Dying Patient Receive Baptism

Description of the client's circumstances and the spiritual care offered:

An elderly male patient in respiratory failure had been in ICU for 15 days when the chaplain was called. The patient had a "Do Not Resuscitate" (DNR) order in place. All machines except for oxygen, an IV, and monitoring equipment had been removed. The doctor and nurses had recently told the family that it would not be long.

The family was concerned that the patient, though willing, had not been baptized by immersion because of a disability that prevented him from entering the baptismal pool. The patient's family wanted to know if the chaplain could baptize the patient. The chaplain worked out a compromise with the family, with the nurse's okay: immersion was not feasible, but pouring water upon the patient's head, hands, and feet could be done. The family agreed, and *the patient was indeed baptized* in that way, with the family—who had strongly affirmed the patient's deep faith and spiritual mentoring—responding on the patient's behalf to the questions read from the *United Methodist Book of Worship*. The patient roused and seemed to understand the significance of the pouring. It was a time of tearful appreciation by all.

Description of what the practitioner, upon reflection, considers most appropriate:

The chaplain could have encouraged the lead family member to more completely articulate the family's faith and the patient's own faith journey, so as to better understand their concept of baptism and how they might interpret the ritual performed.

Fear of Death near End of Life

Description of the client's circumstances and the spiritual care offered:

The chaplain received a page from an LPN at a long-term care facility who said a patient had requested a chaplain. The chaplain asked if anything in particular was happening. The LPN said the patient was very anxious. Upon her arrival, the chaplain was greeted by another LPN, who stated that the referring LPN was busy and that she would take the chaplain to the patient. She quickly led the chaplain to the hallway, stopped, and pointed. "There she is: the woman in the doorway clutching her Bible." An elderly woman in a wheelchair made eye contact with the chaplain, who then gave a smile of acknowledgment. The patient rolled backward into her room, inviting the chaplain in.

The patient told the chaplain, "I just feel so anxious." The patient had a tremor in her hands and arms, although it was not obvious if this was a physical impairment or a result of anxiety. Her breathing was labored as though she had been running. The chaplain led the patient through a few relaxation exercises, suggesting that she close her eyes. She refused, saying, "I don't want to close my eyes."

The chaplain asked, "What happens when you close your eyes?" Further inquiry revealed the patient was concerned that she would fall asleep and perhaps die. She had been having dreams of dying, which to her meant that she would not get to see her grandchildren grow up. She shared her perception that the doctor and her children had neglected to visit her, and stated that she felt claustrophobic in her current room.

The chaplain explored the patient's faith resources and learned she had a Pentecostal background. The patient said, "I cry out to God all the time. It doesn't do any good." She showed the chaplain her Bible, which fell open to Psalm 23. The chaplain, believing that the patient's spiritual issue was feeling abandoned by God, family, and doctor, shared a verse from Psalm 22: "My God, my God, why have you forsaken me?" The chaplain prayed with the patient for relief from her anxiety and also encouraged her to pray, *which she did.*

"*I feel better now,*" the patient said, and then continued, "I'm never going to go home." The chaplain told the patient that she would check to see if the doctor could come soon. When she did, the LPN told the chaplain that the doctor had just seen the patient and that she often refused her medications—she had renal disease and was on dialysis. Her son came frequently and the patient spoke with her children daily on the phone. The chaplain returned to the patient and encouraged her to take her medications to help her get better. The patient agreed that she *would like the unit chaplain to see her soon.*

Description of what the practitioner, upon reflection,
considers most appropriate:

First, the chaplain would have inquired with the nurse prior to
the visit about the circumstances creating the patient's anxiety.
Since the patient was in a long-term care facility, it would have
been helpful to ask how this patient was fitting into the home and
how the staff felt about this patient.

Second, the chaplain did not realize that the patient was indeed
facing possible death. So the spiritual assessment was perceived
to be abandonment by God and family when it was more likely
"fear of death near end of life." Ideally, the chaplain would have
journeyed with the patient longer before proposing an intervention. The chaplain could have asked the patient to share more
about her dreams. This would give insight regarding the type of
fear with which the patient was struggling.

Lastly, the chaplain would ideally have followed the patient's
reference to Psalm 23 by asking, "What does Psalm 23 mean to
you?" The reference to "walking through the valley of the shad-
ow of death" may have been most relevant. The chaplain would
not have needed to concern herself with the medical treatment
other than to inquire with the nurse as to nature of the patient's
care, nor have especially needed to speak to the patient about
compliance.

Background information that the practitioner considers useful:

Ira Byock, *Dying Well: The Prospect for Growth at the End of Life.* New
    York: Riverhead, 1997.
Sherwin B. Nuland, *How We Die: Reflections on Life's Final Chapter.* New
    York: Knopf, 1994.

Fetal Demise, with Nominal Catholic Parents Requesting a Bedside Service

A description of the patient's circumstances
and the spiritual care offered:

The patient was aware that her infant was not alive in her womb. She was waiting for her water to break to receive her child. The patient had been informed that this would be three to four hours away. Present in the room were her husband, the husband's best friend, and a six-year-old niece. The problems were how to address the intimate feelings and needs of the patient in the presence of a group diverse in age, relationship, and spiritual needs. Though the patient was uncomfortable in a church setting, both she and the husband *requested a prayer service* in her hospital room (with the stillborn child in her arms). A brief *service of prayer was held.*

A description of what the practitioner, upon reflection,
considers most appropriate:

If the chaplain were in a similar situation again, the chaplain would explain options more carefully. Prayer is an important element in this process, but the mother's feelings and thoughts might not have embraced God's love at the time.

Background information that the practitioner considers useful:

Kate Caelli, Jill Downie, and Angeline Letendre, "Parents' Experiences of Midwife-Managed Care Following the Loss of a Baby in a Previous Pregnancy." *Journal of Advanced Nursing* 39:2, July 2002. 127–136.

"Family Pediatrics: Report of the Task Force on the Family." *Pediatrics* 111: supplement 2, June 2003. 1541–1571.

"Meeting the Needs of Parents around the Time of Diagnosis of Disability among Their Children." *Pediatrics* 114:4, October 2004. e477–e482.

Intuitive Caregiving during Terminal Illness

Description of the client's circumstances
and the spiritual care offered:

A married couple, residents of a retirement community, attended chapel services regularly. The recently hired and untrained chaplain became acquainted with them and even attended their anniversary celebration. As the wife's health declined, her three daughters began to visit more regularly. The end drew near, and the chaplain began to wonder if the resident was even aware of her pastoral presence and prayers.

One Sunday one of the daughters brought her mother to the ward's worship along with two grandchildren. The chaplain invited them to read Scripture in worship, and a granddaughter accepted the invitation. The family *expressed gratitude* for her participation, a memory they later indicated that they would especially cherish because the resident died the next week.

The chaplain *conducted a memorial service* for the deceased resident in the community chapel and worked with the family to celebrate her life on that occasion.

Description of what the practitioner, upon reflection,
considers most appropriate:

The chaplain reflected later that with minimal training she would not have been as timid during her visits. She stated that she would have approached the one needing care as though the resident understood everything she was communicating (especially Scripture passages and prayer). In addition, she would have been more proactive in communicating with family members when they came to visit their mother.

Background information that the practitioner considers useful:

William A. Clebsch and Charles R. Jaekle, *Pastoral Care in Historical Perspective*. New York: Jason Aronson, 1994.
John J. Gleason Jr., *Growing Up to God*. Nashville: Abingdon, 1975.

Lawrence E. Holst, ed., *Hospital Ministry: The Role of the Chaplain Today.* New York: Wipf & Stock, 2007.

Larry VandeCreek and Arthur M. Lucas, eds., *The Discipline for Pastoral Care Giving.* Binghamton: Haworth, 2001.

Lamenting Terminal Cancer Patient

Description of the client's circumstances
and the spiritual care offered:

A 58-year-old nominally Catholic, divorced mother of two was a hospice inpatient. She suffered from metastasized breast cancer that affected her motor abilities, and her radiation treatment had left her bald. She was cared for by her mother, who had not accepted her daughter's dying and therefore did not want to fully address end-of-life issues. The patient's ex-husband lived out of state with one child; the other child was incarcerated. The patient had an uncertain relationship with her boyfriend.

Recently, in her first contact with a priest in a long time, the patient had received the Sacrament of the Sick. She believed God could provide a miracle and return some of her motor ability. Since that had not happened, she believed she had done something (or not done something) to contribute to this. She was concerned that she had not been grateful enough and reasoned that that was why God was not healing her.

Having repeated her distress to the hospice nurse, social worker, and hospice aide, the patient did so once again with the chaplain. In his third visit, he read from Psalm 139: "O LORD, you have searched me and known me. . . . I come to the end—I am still with you." The patient responded, "*That was beautiful.*" He also read Psalm 19 and tied it to the suffering of Christ.

However, she couldn't quite connect, and the chaplain sensed her tiredness. With her permission, he prayed, "God, we come before you with deep needs. (Patient) has such hurt and pain right now, and she, like your Son, Jesus, cries out to you from her place of suffering. You see her; you know her life, her heart, her tears.

May she know your comfort and power. In your name, amen."
He then took his leave.

Description of what the practitioner, upon reflection, considers most appropriate:

In retrospect the chaplain wrote: "[I] spoke to the patient about the place of lament in Scriptures without giving her the opportunity to voice her own lament." In fairness, the chaplain did seem to allow, and even encourage, her to do so, and only brought the conversation to a close because he was sensitive to her exhaustion. He could have further ministered by continuing to help the patient express her lament and, importantly, help her feel heard.

The use of laments from the patient's own faith tradition might also have been beneficial, and the chaplain could have invited the patient to enter into them herself by asking if selections voiced her feelings. The chaplain could also have provided education, support, and encouragement to all other members of the treatment team, helping them use their own active listening skills in order to add to the patient's experience of being heard. This would have reduced the patient's feelings of isolation and created space in the patient's life for God's healing presence to be felt.

Several appropriate communication strategies would be to name the suffering, identify the losses, relieve isolation, shift perception, empower, support faith, support the best self, introduce hope, and appropriate touch. (See reference below.)

Background information that the practitioner considers useful:

B. Bub, "The Patient's Lament: Hidden Key to Effective Communication," *Medical Humanities* 30:2, December 2004, 63–69.

Long-Term Dialysis Patient Nearing Death

Description of the client's circumstances and the spiritual care offered:

A professing Christian believer, active congregation member, and grandmother who lived a life guided by faith had long-term health issues. These issues led to kidney dialysis more than three times per week for an extended time. The dialysis had become ineffective in stabilizing her situation and caused greater pain overall. She had a growing conviction that she should discontinue the now-ineffective measures and spend whatever time remained as closely and actively as possible with her family living nearby, that they might "walk the last mile together as best as could be."

In a family conference, her minister helped her *verbalize her situation*, her faith, and her desire for family support and time together. This was *well received* and shared among family members, including a son-in-law and two preteen granddaughters.

Description of what the practitioner, upon reflection, considers most appropriate:

Upon reflection the minister would take more time, in as unobtrusive a manner as possible, to follow up with the family. Perhaps the minister would arrange one or two meetings for the family to share their feelings and faith with one another. The meetings could also provide the family opportunities to pray with and for one another, in view of the days and years ahead, as believers within the family unit.

Managing a Large Family during a Pediatric Unit Code Blue

Description of the client's circumstances
and the spiritual care offered:

The chaplain was called to a Code Blue (resuscitation required) on the pediatric unit. He spent time with family (more than 30 people) and with staff, mostly as a quiet presence, and offered prayer with the grandparents. The child was transferred to the ER for transport by air to another hospital, but the child later died.

At that point, the chaplain spent time with the father and grandparents. The child's mother was very angry and distraught and did not want anything to do with religious things. A time of prayer with the father ensued when he responded to the chaplain's body language—*hands folded in a prayerful attitude.*

Description of what the practitioner, upon reflection,
considers most appropriate:

The intervention with the family seemed satisfactory. However, in a similar situation the chaplain would understand the intervention to have just begun, both for staff and for him as pastoral caregiver. He would attend the debriefing with the Employee Assistance Program representative, and would provide ongoing pastoral care for staff. Finally, he would attend to self-care, especially regarding feelings of helplessness and emotional involvement.

Matter-of-Fact Acceptance of Terminal Illness

Description of the client's circumstances
and the spiritual care offered:

The chaplain arrived at the room of a 48-year-old male cancer patient to conduct a spiritual assessment and found him with his wife seated beside him. Although taken aback at first by the scar tissue in the patient's eye socket, the chaplain greeted them both, introduced himself and the purpose of his visit, and asked about the patient's situation. The patient stated very plainly his condition and medical prognosis. He was "full of cancer," and it had initially begun as colon and prostate cancer. He said he could do nothing about his condition at this point and that he had accepted it.

The patient spoke in a matter-of-fact voice, with very little emotional affect. He appeared resigned to what was going to happen and expressed very few regrets about his life. When asked whether he had given thought to the end of his life, he said he had indeed, and again stated that he couldn't change things, that he had done what he could and could do nothing more. This was said with a finality that seemed to express acceptance of his impending death. The patient was to be discharged late that same day.

The chaplain learned that the patient and his wife had two 20-something sons and an 18-month-old granddaughter. They had recently begun attending a local Baptist church, and the patient indicated that the members knew of his being in the hospital. At that point, the chaplain asked if he could say a prayer. Both responded in the affirmative. He prayed, "Dear Lord, I pray for (Patient and Wife) during this really tough time. I ask that you would give them strength and courage. I pray for (Patient), that you would show him your purposes for him even now. Give him the strength to go through this time and to take care of the things that he feels he needs to do. I pray in your name, amen."

The patient *thanked him* with *tears in his eyes*. The chaplain took his leave after explaining follow-up chaplaincy services and giving the patient his card.

Description of what the practitioner, upon reflection, considers most appropriate:

The chaplain's own experience of similar illness gave him a special sensitivity to the patient's situation. Thus, he was prepared to "walk beside the patient" and was able to explore with the patient his attitude and feelings toward impending death: seeming acceptance with minimal emotion, except for tears during the prayer.

In retrospect the chaplain could perhaps have attempted to bring the patient's wife into the conversation regarding her own feelings, although she seemed reticent throughout the visit except to "beam" at the mention of the granddaughter.

Background information that the practitioner considers useful:

Jan Selliken, Bernard and Miriam Schneider, *The True Work of Dying: A Practical and Compassionate Guide to Easing the Dying Process.* New York: Avon, 1996.

Mother Coping with Daughter's End-Stage Cancer Diagnosis

Description of the client's circumstances
and the spiritual care offered:

The Protestant chaplain was paged to the bedside of a medicated and drowsy 26-year-old female to attend to her mother. The patient was a non-practicing Jew, and her mother was unaffiliated with a synagogue as well. The mother was having difficulty coping with the end-stage cancer diagnosis that had been given to her daughter.

During several visits, the chaplain provided active listening, prayer, and gentle guided imagery as he bore witness to the mother's sorrow. He was able to establish trust with these efforts in addition to his willingness simply to be with her as she *lamented* and *raised the "why" questions* regarding mortality, love, and the existence of God.

After these visits had concluded, the patient's mother *wrote a highly complimentary letter* to the hospital CEO regarding the chaplain's ministry.

Description of what the practitioner, upon reflection, considers most appropriate:

The chaplain's considerable knowledge of her religious tradition—gathered in part from living in an area with a high Jewish population, in part from his reading, and in part from associating with local rabbis—had contributed to meeting the mother's intellectual needs as she processed such painful information and anticipated a life without her daughter.

In retrospect the chaplain felt that he would not have done much differently. He cited his motto in emphasizing the effectiveness of listening more than talking: "Two eyes, two ears, [only] one mouth." The mother's letter to the CEO validated the effectiveness of the chaplain's ministry.

However, an area for exploration in a similar situation would be to gently probe beyond the intellectual content to determine whether it masked feelings in need of healing release.

Multiple Issues at the End of Life

Description of the client's circumstances and the spiritual care offered:

The hospice chaplain did an assessment with a 60-year-old married male patient with stepchildren. He was a Vietnam veteran with PTSD, Agent Orange aftereffects, metastasized lung cancer, and alcohol dependence. His wife was a former RN who was affectively engaged (with high anxiety) in the interview, noting that this would be her second husband lost to death. The family was strongly Pentecostal and poor but not destitute.

In the first encounter, after the chaplain asked the wife to give him time alone with the patient, the patient admitted that she often spoke for him instead of letting him speak for himself. The patient also said his wife disagreed with his desire to be cremated. Furthermore, he noted that throughout their married life his wife would take him on trips against his will.

The patient *confided* to the chaplain that every time he tried to "do better," he would "hit a wall." Following further discussion, which allowed the patient to share his difficulties and bring his faith background to light, the chaplain sensed "a leading of the Spirit." He suggested that the wall the patient was hitting was "the cross," and that he look up Colossians 3:1-3, which reads: "So if you have been raised with Christ, seek the things that are above, where Christ is, seated at the right hand of God. Set your minds on things that are above, not on things that are on earth, for you have died, and your life is hidden with Christ in God." These words seemed to *manifest peace* upon the patient. He *recalled this* passage in each successive visit, while pointing upward, and never spoke again of his frustration with the wall.

Later the chaplain shared at the patient's funeral.

Description of what the practitioner, upon reflection, considers most appropriate:

In retrospect the chaplain might have asked for a more private conversation with the patient, or asked the patient to say more about his "wall" in spiritual terms, or offered a biblical prescription. Otherwise the chaplain felt that he would not have proceeded much differently.

Background information that the practitioner considers useful:

Deborah Howard, *Sunsets: Reflections for Life's Final Journey*. Wheaton: Crossway, 2005.

Nonreligious Husband in Shock at Wife's Death

Description of the client's circumstances and the spiritual care offered:

The chaplain was paged to the ER at 6:30 a.m. to attend to a death. When she arrived at the nurses' station, she was informed by the attending nurse that the patient had died of cardiac arrest after being transported from an assisted living facility. The chaplain was further told that the husband of the woman was in the room with the body. The nurse reported that she had offered the man spiritual care assistance, but he had declined, stating his bias against religious matters.

In the course of the chaplain's conversation with the husband, the man indicated that he was not prepared to see his wife die, despite her life-threatening condition. In recounting the discovery that morning that he could not wake his wife, he reported "hitting the panic button." The chaplain replied, "So even though she had breathing problems, you weren't ready for this to happen?" The husband acknowledged this was true and *described both his and his wife's choices* to deny the impending death.

The chaplain discovered that the couple had been married for 63 years, and the husband went on to *recount his memory* of their meeting for the first time, moving him to *tears* and other expressions of grief. The chaplain offered to pray, and the husband passively agreed.

Description of what the practitioner, upon reflection, considers most appropriate:

The chaplain was able to join the husband in the midst of his overwhelming grief, as evidenced by enabling him to tell his story and achieve some catharsis despite his resistance to "religious" things and persons.

The catharsis might have been made easier with more empathic observations of feelings, such as, "That must have been so hard—a truly frightening moment." Such responses could have helped the husband better realize he had been heard and emotionally validated in his shock and grief, so that he could more fully experience comfort and healing. An additional intervention would have been to invite him to continue the story regarding his marriage, so as to keep him in a mood of remembrance that would expedite his grief process.

Background information that the practitioner considers useful:

Richard Dana, Lewis Bernstein, and Rosalyn S. Bernstein, "The Reassuring Response," *Interviewing: A Guide for Health Professionals.* New York: Appleton-Century Crofts, 1985.

Panicked Spouse of a New Hospice Patient

Description of the client's circumstances and the spiritual care offered:

The male patient, in his middle years, was a direct admission (not previously a hospice patient but coming directly from home or hospital), indicating a fast-moving illness. The patient's nurse and a daughter had previously indicated to the chaplain that the patient's wife was emotionally distraught.

In the chaplain's second visit, with a different daughter present, the wife's opening statement was that she was "miserable." The wife *shared* that: (1) they were moving to this area and had just closed on a house; (2) they had left family and friends behind; (3) they had plans for their future together; (4) this diagnosis and prognosis came swiftly and suddenly; and (5) now she was feeling very alone. The daughter assured her mother that she would be able to move back to their previous location where she would again have the close support of her family, friends, and church community.

The wife began to shake and complain of being cold. A blanket was wrapped around her shoulders and a cup of coffee was brought to her. She began to heave as if nauseated, and the chaplain found a nurse to assist her. It was decided that she needed to go get some rest, and she left with a newly arrived friend of the family. After their departure, the chaplain spoke briefly with the daughter and then excused himself because he was feeling shaken by the incident.

Description of what the practitioner, upon reflection, considers most appropriate:

In general the chaplain would have prepared for the possibility of acute distress in any patient, family member, or staff person. Specifically, the patient's spouse, daughter, and the chaplain would have had a conversation that encouraged the spouse to fully share her grief without anyone being too quick to mention positive outcomes. Following the exit of the upset spouse and after the chaplain had composed himself, he would have returned to further converse with the daughter about how she was doing and how to plan for follow-up with her mother.

Background information that the practitioner considers useful:

Wayne E. Oates, *The Minister's Own Mental Health*. New York: Channel, 1961.

Rectifying a Mistaken Cremation

Description of the client's circumstances and the spiritual care offered:

The hospital chaplain was called to the laboratory to assist with a dilemma. A stillborn baby had been taken for a postmortem, and the pathologist mistakenly cremated the baby per the standard practice in his past employment. The parents had wanted to bury the baby instead. The chaplain agreed that the parents needed to be told immediately that there had been a mistake, but that every effort would be made to rectify it so that they could still be able to have a graveside service. The chaplain went with the pathologist for support while he explained his error.

The chaplain found and purchased a porcelain container for the cremains. The container was blue (the baby was male) and had red and yellow flowers on the side. The chaplain also had a matching floral arrangement made. The pathologist was able to gather the cremains together, and the maintenance department was able to glue the lid closed. Later that afternoon the staff was able to present the family with the way they had resolved this, and the *chaplain was able to provide a brief service and memorial prayer at the bedside* when staff gave the family the ashes and flowers.

Description of what the practitioner, upon reflection, considers most appropriate:

The family felt that staff members had gone beyond what they had expected and were grateful for the effort put into correcting the mistake. Thus, the intervention was considered a success.

Background information that the practitioner considers useful:

Luke 6:31

Saying Good-bye to a Loved One

Description of the client's circumstances and the spiritual care offered:

The minister, a local clergy volunteer, was called into the hospital for a death in the ICU at 3:30 a.m. An 88-year-old woman had been admitted only 30 minutes prior from the ER and had suddenly died.

The minister met with her two children initially, whom he learned had been providing extensive care for her as her health had deteriorated over time. The minister helped them process her death, including saying good-bye to their mother, and facilitated their sharing about their mother when all the family had gathered.

The minister was careful not to dominate the conversation, allowing them to share about their mother and continue their memory-making process. At one point, he did note that it would be a blessed relief to no longer continue their caring but taxing routine of having a family member constantly present with her, to which they *responded with sad but relieved agreement.*

He led them in prayer to conclude the visit. As he left, the family *expressed their gratitude* for his coming out to be with them in the middle of the night.

Description of what the practitioner, upon reflection, considers most appropriate:

In retrospect the minister felt he had provided adequate support. However, he would have especially invited the RN to join the family circle in the final prayer, even though she was present on the periphery.

Simultaneous Ministries to Dying Patient and Loved One

Description of the client's circumstances and the spiritual care offered:

The chaplain received a referral from an LPN in a long-term rehabilitation center for a 59-year-old female patient. The LPN said, "She's in hospice and I think she is close to the time." As the chaplain entered the patient's room, she saw two women: a daughter-in-law and a friend of the family. The patient appeared to be sleeping. The chaplain began to speak with the daughter-in-law at the side of the bed and then noticed that the patient was awake and looking at the chaplain. The chaplain moved to the patient's bedside.

The patient asked the chaplain to call her pastor and the hospice chaplain. The daughter-in-law interjected that it was a Nazarene pastor, and that both clergy had been there. The chaplain assumed that the patient was disoriented and that the pastors had visited recently. The chaplain placed her hand on top of the patient's left hand, which was resting on her chest. The patient made eye contact and then closed her eyes. The chaplain remarked, "You feel at peace." *"Yes," said the patient, ". . . at peace. I'm ready."* The chaplain replied, "You're ready to go. . . . You are ready to meet Jesus." At that point, the patient fell into such a deep sleep that the chaplain wondered for a moment if she had died. The chaplain gently removed her hand from the patient's and sat by the daughter-in-law.

The daughter-in-law commented, "She *is* ready. She has been ready for a while. I'm not sure why she is still here." The chaplain inquired if the patient had been able to say good-bye to everyone. Only a niece and nephew had not spoken with her and probably would not be coming. The daughter-in-law spoke of her observation of the patient's decline and said, "I keep thinking that if I stay with her I'll see Jesus come to take her." The chaplain encouraged her to talk more and led her into *life review*. The daughter-in-law said, "She means so much to me. She became my mom when mine died. She only had sons, and told me I was the daughter she never had."

The daughter-in-law requested prayer for her husband. The chaplain prayed, "Dear loving God, thank you for sharing (Patient) with us. Her life was a loving example. She said she is ready to go home. Please help make this last part of her journey go smoothly with little pain. Bless (Daughter-in-law) and her husband with peace and patience as they say their good-byes, knowing they will always have (Patient) in their hearts. Thank you for being with us always, we pray, amen." The daughter-in-law *thanked* the chaplain for her prayer and visit.

Description of what the practitioner, upon reflection, considers most appropriate:

In a more ideal visit, the chaplain would have asked the LPN why she believed the patient needed care. The chaplain would have made the patient the primary focus of the visit (giving a helpless, dying person value), perhaps asking the daughter-in-law for time alone with the patient. This would honor the patient, giving her the ability to ask for what she needed without the daughter-in-law speaking for her.

The chaplain would also try to recognize the family system dynamics more fully. If the daughter-in-law wanted to speak with the chaplain, it would have been best to speak outside the room so that the patient would not overhear comments such as, "I don't know why she is still here." The chaplain would have clarified when the pastor and chaplain had last visited and contacted them on behalf of the patient if they had not recently attended.

Background information that the practitioner considers useful:

Ira Byock, *Dying Well: The Prospect for Growth at the End of Life.* New York: Riverhead, 1997. 217–239.

Sherwin B. Nuland, *How We Die: Reflections on Life's Final Chapter.* New York: Alfred A. Knopf, 1993. 242–262.

Stephen B. Roberts, ed., *Professional Spiritual and Pastoral Care: A Practical Clergy and Chaplain's Handbook.* Woodstock, VT: SkyLight Paths, 2012. 149–161.

Slowly Dying Mother

Description of the client's circumstances and the spiritual care offered:

The chaplain had visited with the daughter of a hospice patient on the daughter's previous visits from the northeastern United States to her mother's hospice in the South. At this point the daughter was trying to decide whether to fly home for a few days to attend to her children and husband after three days with her mother. The daughter had *shared* with the chaplain that her relationship with her mother had not always been easy. Furthermore, on the day before this encounter, the mother had reversed her decision regarding receiving the Sacrament of the Sick. While the patient was busy with staff and other visitors waited, the chaplain sat with the daughter and her mother's healthcare surrogate, who dominated the conversation.

Description of what the practitioner, upon reflection, considers most appropriate:

The chaplain could have invited the daughter to reflect on her feelings instead of focusing on options. More appropriate interventions might have been: "I hear it is a hard decision," or "My sense is that you want to stay," or "Sometimes we don't know what to do," or "It's a dilemma."

As the chaplain became aware that the healthcare surrogate was dominating the conversation, she could have invited the daughter to step out and walk down the hall with her while the patient was busy. While alone with the daughter, the chaplain could have learned more about the patient's decision not to receive the Sacrament of the Sick, and could have continued to help the daughter process her feelings and options.

Timing Visits with the Family of a Dying Patient

Description of the client's circumstances
and the spiritual care offered:

A hospice patient in her fifties was on vacation with her family when she became unresponsive and was brought to the ER. The chaplain went to the ER waiting room to support the patient's family and, in particular, the daughter. However, other staff interrupted the pastoral visit numerous times. The daughter was also making and receiving many phone calls. The chaplain thought it best to return later.

After several hours passed, the chaplain returned to visit the daughter and other family members. The patient had died shortly before his arrival; the family was still present. The chaplain again offered support to the daughter and family but mostly focused on providing support to the daughter. An offer of prayer was made, but the family declined due to the patient's own religious beliefs. However, the chaplain was able to establish rapport with the family based on the family's concerns about the patient's beliefs. Shortly afterward, the family *thanked* the chaplain and left the hospital.

Description of what the practitioner, upon reflection,
considers most appropriate:

Ideally, the chaplain would have offered support to all family
members early on, rather than to just one member, and would
have made frequent brief visits rather than one long visit. Shorter
visits would mesh better with the family members' involvement
with a number of other matters. In addition, shorter and more
frequent visits would have provided a continuity of pastoral
presence and more opportunities for family members to feel supported, especially for vacationers away from their normal sur-
roundings and other family members.

Background information that the practitioner considers useful:

Therese A. Rando, *Grief, Dying, and Death: Clinical Interventions for
Caregivers.* Champaign, IL: Research Press, 1984.

Two Simultaneous ICU Deathbed Situations

Description of the client's circumstances
and the spiritual care offered:

The only chaplain on duty arrived at the ICU to make her rounds
and learned from the charge nurse that two patients were dying.
The first was a 95-year-old woman whose family was on the way
and well prepared to sign for Comfort Measures Only (CMO)
status. The other was a 54-year-old homeless man. His sister had
been located and was on her way to see him and to sign for CMO
status also. The chaplain went to each room and offered a short
blessing. After finishing at the man's room, she learned that the
woman's family had arrived and was asking for the chaplain.

After asking to be informed when the man's sister had arrived,
the chaplain visited with the woman's family as they *shared* loving stories, Scripture readings, and prayers. As she concluded, the
other patient's nurse alerted the chaplain to the sister's arrival.
The chaplain turned back to the woman's family to explain that
she was needed across the unit and would be available later if

they needed her. The family *expressed their gratitude*, and one member offered the chaplain a blessing and prayer for the other patient.

Although less than five minutes had elapsed, the man's sister had already left, leaving the dying patient alone. The chaplain remained with the male patient, offering prayers, speaking to him, and stroking his arm and hair. As she left, the chaplain asked his nurse to alert her before the extubation was to take place. That occurred within an hour, and the chaplain remained, speaking, reflecting, and praying a prayer of commemoration as the man drew his last breath. The nurse *thanked* the chaplain for being there, thereby allowing the nurse to tend to her other critical patient. The chaplain checked on the woman's family and left the unit.

Description of what the practitioner, upon reflection, considers most appropriate:

Ideally, the chaplain would have met with the homeless patient's sister to offer comfort, support, and condolences. Since both deaths were occurring within the same unit, navigation between the two rooms was unhampered. In addition, the relationship between the chaplain and nursing staff was well established, easing the movements and trust between them. Since there were no other crises or codes during that time, the chaplain was able to be available so that no patient would die alone.

Background information that the practitioner considers useful:

Agnes Sanford, ed., *The Healing Light*. Toronto: Macalester Park, 1972.

Wife of a Dying Spouse

Description of the client's circumstances and the spiritual care offered:

In the room of a nonresponsive, dying male patient, his wife, her sister, and a nurse were in conversation when the chaplain arrived. In the wife's initial statement to the chaplain, she said, "They are right. I can't keep this up anymore." Her sister explained her view that the wife needed to take better care of herself and added that the patient was holding on because he didn't want to leave his wife. The wife *explained her frustration*: that she had indeed given the patient permission to "go and be in heaven," but that his children were praying that he would not die. She felt the children seemed neither to understand the disease's progression nor appreciate their father's lack of quality of life.

The chaplain offered the scriptural account of the apostle Paul, citing Paul's own struggle with the desire to go and be with God vis-à-vis staying alive for the benefit of the Philippian church (Philippians 1:22-24).

A nurse interrupted the visit to apply a medical patch to the patient. Following the interruption, the wife requested prayer, and after the prayer the chaplain left.

Description of what the practitioner, upon reflection, considers most appropriate:

Ideally, the chaplain would have tried to help the wife better hold in tension the importance of her presence at her husband's bedside and her own need for respite care, again using the example of the apostle Paul. In so doing, the chaplain would also have sought more appreciation for the children's inability to be present during their father's last hours.

Moreover, the chaplain would have invited the wife to share more of her own experience in the patient's dying process. After the nursing interruption and perhaps before the prayer, the chaplain would have offered to continue addressing the wife's concerns if she so chose, or if not, to bless her desire to leave and get some rest.

Background information that the practitioner considers useful:

Cynthia Pearson and Margaret Stubbs, *Parting Company: Understanding the Loss of a Loved One—The Caregiver's Journey.* Seattle: Seal, 1999.

Ministry in Psycho-Spiritual Crises

As noted in the introduction to Section One, the term *crisis* is generally understood to be the experience of distress caused by a disruption in the balancing mechanisms that govern our daily lives. In this section, this disruption is caused by the anticipation or reality that this delicate balance cannot be maintained, but mostly for *non*physical reasons.

Thus, a psycho-spiritual crisis can be best understood as the impact of an actual or anticipated loss (or even gain), in which we are forced to deal with the change in ways very different from our usual patterns of response. If not too overwhelming, such crises can become teachable moments. May you find in these 46 case descriptions ideas to apply as you minister to those in psycho-spiritual crises, and may your learning spur you toward the most redemptive possible new response patterns.

Anger after Attempted Suicide

**Description of the client's circumstances
and the spiritual care offered:**

Immediately after the chaplain introduced himself, the female patient, who had survived a suicide attempt, *began to weep*. She cried throughout the visit. She *expressed anger* with her husband and "other things," saying, "Yes, I took some pills . . . because I was angry with my husband and [because] there's a lot of stuff going on in my life . . . [and] because I wanted to die."

With the chaplain interspersing supportive and active listening comments, other excerpts of their encounter included these statements: "Yes, I just needed an escape from the pressure of everything. I've had to deal with a lot before and I was able to deal with it, but this time I wasn't able to do it. . . . I really don't want to be here. . . . My husband brought me in here. . . . Yes, it has been hard; there's so much on my mind, and being here, all I have time to do is think about everything. . . . I'm *feeling broken*. . . ." She was quiet for a few moments, *continuing to shed tears*. "I don't know. It's just hard." The interview concluded with prayer.

**Description of what the practitioner, upon reflection,
considers most appropriate:**

The chaplain sought to provide a ministry of listening presence and support to enable some life review in addition to prayer. The patient's spiritual issues and needs included coping, anger, feelings of helplessness, and feelings of hopelessness after her attempted suicide. Examples of the chaplain's interventions included "I hear that you are angry. Can you tell me more about your anger?" "Sounds like the anger is difficult for you." "What is the anger about?" and "Why are you angry with your husband?" These responsive questions allowed the patient to explore her anger to a measured extent.

Background information that the practitioner considers useful:

Janet Malone, "Exploring Human Anger," *Human Development* 15:1, Spring 1994. 33–38.

Anger at Dying Husband

Description of the client's circumstances and the spiritual care offered:

The male patient was in hospice, being cared for at home, and was still alert. He had good support from his church and especially from the men's Bible study group and ushers group. Prior to the visit, the chaplain had been forewarned by the social worker about the patient's stormy marriage, so when making her visit, the chaplain told the wife she would like to talk with the spouses separately.

The man acknowledged a poor relationship with his wife, stating that he was a workaholic. He also admitted having a very broken relationship with one of his sons. The husband *expressed guilt* about his verbal abuse of the wife but admitted he couldn't control himself well. Forgiveness was explored. He did not express a desire for amends with the son he had not seen in over a year. The patient said work was his job and his play and his satisfaction. He had no regrets about life choices. He *requested prayer* for forgiveness from God as well as ability to be kinder to his wife as she cared for him.

With the wife the chaplain mostly listened as she *cried* and *talked* about the misery of her life and marriage. The wife "hated" her husband of 50 years and always had, because he was so verbally abusive to her. She attended a church, not her husband's, because she did not feel support at her husband's church. Her church of the most recent months was "a better place" for her. She would not divorce because of the promise she made to her spouse and God years ago. She also had no relationship with the estranged son, and was closer to the disabled son who lived states away.

A couple of days after the visit, the wife called the chaplain, angry with her husband's pastor who had come to visit at the chaplain's and husband's request. The pastor had not been visiting the patient up to that point. She confronted the pastor about his absence, to which the pastor replied, "(Patient) has had many visits from men of the church." She said that was not the same as visits from the pastor, so the pastor left. The chaplain listened to the wife, acknowledged her frustration, but said now the wife would need to figure out how to leave this behind or she would live in more pain. Asked how she might lower her expectations or aim to forgive, the wife said she knew she needed to forgive. The chaplain suggested a book about grace as a helpful resource toward that goal.

At the time of this phone call, the husband was in a coma.

Description of what the practitioner, upon reflection, considers most appropriate:

As a hospice chaplain, the chaplain "would change the frequency of [her] visits to weekly if at all possible." (Standard frequency in her hospice was once per month.) The chaplain did considerable phone collaboration with the hospice RN and social worker in order for all of them to support the family in a unified manner.

Background information that the practitioner considers useful:

Donald B. Kraybill, Steven M. Nolt, and David L. Weaver, *Amish Grace*. Hoboken, NJ: John Wiley & Sons, 2010.
Matthew 6:14-15; 18:21-22; Ephesians 4:31-32; Colossians 3:13

Angry, Feeling Betrayed and Powerless

Description of the client's circumstances
and the spiritual care offered:

A 73-year-old retired male was brought to the hospital by his daughter and found himself admitted there and unable to return home.

The chaplain invited the patient to verbalize his feelings of anger and frustration, and to share his story. The patient *shared* about his law practice, his aviation experiences, boating, and horses. He had pictures of these interests on his wall.

The chaplain invited the patient to consider: if a genie could grant him a wish, what would he ask for? He answered, "Go back to my home!" By this point, the patient was *more relaxed* and *smiling*.

The chaplain concluded the conversation with his hope and prayer that the Lord would guide the patient in finding the most realistic way to move forward with his life.

Description of what the practitioner, upon reflection,
considers most appropriate:

In retrospect the chaplain would still have invited the patient to verbalize his feelings of anger, but this time he would ask the patient to be more specific: anger against God, his daughter, etc. The patient had the most trouble recognizing that he was dying and could not go back to his own house, continue drinking, or provide for himself.

Also, the chaplain would strive to meet his own need to be objective and not get entangled in the "victim" feelings of the patient, a lawyer who was articulate in spinning out ideas of conspiracies against him.

Anticipatory Grief and End-of-Life Care to Family Members

Description of the client's circumstances
and the spiritual care offered:

An attending nurse paged the chaplain to visit a family. The doctor had just delivered news that the patient, in her mid-forties and diagnosed with metastasized breast cancer, only had a day or two to live. The news was particularly disturbing because the patient had been recently removed from hospice because of medical improvement.

Upon the chaplain's arrival, she found the patient's husband openly weeping and pleading with the patient to wake up. The patient was unresponsive and coughing. The patient's mother entered a short time later. The chaplain asked questions to gather information about the patient's medical history, the family system, and their faith backgrounds. The husband had no religious affiliation; the mother had a Methodist background; and the patient, according to the mother, "had faith," such that the mother knew "where she [was] going."

There were interruptions by medical staff and family phone calls. Since the mother did not respond to the chaplain's query about whether she preferred the chaplain to stay or give her privacy, the chaplain had difficulty discerning the value of her presence. When she asked the mother at the end of the visit if there was anything else she could do, the mother *requested prayer* and the chaplain prayed.

Then the husband, who had expressed no religious belief and had stated that he had never prayed a day in his life, requested prayer himself when he reentered the room. The chaplain asked how she might pray. *Taking the chaplain's hand*, the husband *tearfully* responded, "I just want her not to be in pain anymore."

The chaplain then prayed, "Dear loving God, we don't understand how and when you heal, but we are asking you to take care of (Patient). Comfort her; make it possible to have relief from her pain. Make your presence known in this room to all who enter. Surround (Patient) and (Husband) and (Mother) and (Nurse) with your peace and love in this painful time. Bless the medical staff with wisdom and loving hands. We give you praise for all the remaining time we have with (Patient). Amen." *Visibly comforted*, the husband *thanked* the chaplain, at which point she took her leave.

Description of what the practitioner, upon reflection, considers most appropriate:

At the technical level, a more effective way of ministering to this husband and mother (or anyone in crisis) might have been to be quietly present without asking so many questions, thereby freeing the chaplain from "fixing" the pain and giving tacit permission for the husband and mother to feel that pain. The chaplain learned that family members may appreciate a calm presence, even if they do not ask the chaplain to stay or do anything specific. If they are sharing personal information with the chaplain, that most likely means the chaplain's presence is desirable.

At a deeper level, this difficult visit culminated in a moving spiritual connection as the husband, who struggled to believe in a loving God, requested prayer for his wife's relief of pain. Some combination of his need, the chaplain's ministrations, and a Presence beyond them both created a few moments of much-needed healing.

Background information that the practitioner considers useful:

Kay Lindahl, *Practicing the Sacred Art of Listening: A Guide to Enrich Your Relationships and Kindle Your Spiritual Life*. Woodstock, VT: SkyLight Paths, 2003.

Howard Stone, *Crisis Counseling*. Minneapolis: Fortress, 1980.

Bad News Harshly Delivered

Description of the client's circumstances
and the spiritual care offered:

The chaplain was asked to meet with a family to offer prayer and support for the outcome of exploratory surgery for a cancerous tumor. He was with the family when the doctor came out to advise the family of the findings. The doctor was blunt and factual, showing little compassion. He stated, "I found cancer and he's going to die." The family asked how long the patient would live, and the doctor replied, "Don't know, and I won't make promises. But he is going to die."

When the doctor left, the family *expressed their outrage* at his harshness, and at the same time felt heartbroken at the news. The chaplain tried to turn their attention in a positive manner to the fact that as long as there is breath, there is hope.

Description of what the practitioner, upon reflection,
considers most appropriate:

The chaplain's effort to lift up hope seemed to help the family keep a more balanced perspective during the next months.

Belated Receipt of a Death Message

Description of the client's circumstances
and the spiritual care offered:

The night chaplain received a referral from the on-call day chaplain. The patient had received some news that was not good, and a visit from the chaplain would be appropriate. The chaplain noted that the name sounded familiar. He had had other conversations with the patient following heart surgery. When the chaplain reached the unit, he stopped at the nurse's station and learned that the patient had just found out that his son had died.

As the chaplain entered the room, the patient was watching television in his chair. He seemed sad. He was wearing his glasses and the lights were off in the room. He had a blanket over him. Early in the conversation, the patient shared that only that morning he found out that his son had died of AIDS the previous week. The chaplain's comment about his angry tone enabled the patient to say that he did not find out about his son's death until a family member called. The son's mother had said that she would inform the patient as soon as it happened but had failed to do so.

After a brief silence the chaplain asked about funeral plans. The patient answered that because of an autopsy, plans were incomplete. He then *vented his frustration* that being in the hospital had kept him from finding out earlier and perhaps even giving him a chance to say one more good-bye. When the chaplain asked about the reason for the information delay, the patient said he did not really know, although he cited the mother's drug and alcohol problems as a possibility. The patient then expressed his exhaustion; the chaplain shared his regrets and made his exit with the patient's *thanks*.

Description of what the practitioner, upon reflection, considers most appropriate:

After the visit, the chaplain had several insights that could have led to a more effective intervention: (1) he could have been less focused on facts toward fixing the patient's problems and instead been more emotionally present; (2) he could have made better use of the silences by letting them run a little longer; and (3) he later realized that some of his assumptions about AIDS were false and these assumptions skewed his responses.

Background information that the practitioner considers useful:

Ernest E. Bruder, *Ministering to Deeply Troubled People*. Englewood Cliffs, NJ: Prentice-Hall, 1963.

Complicated Grief

Description of the client's circumstances
and the spiritual care offered:

The unemployed male patient *immediately got into his story* upon the chaplain's arrival. "I've had some bad news. My mother committed suicide two days ago." Taken aback, the chaplain asked, "Is your father in your life?" to which the patient responded, "My mother shot and killed him," adding, "I was in a coma for three weeks."

At the chaplain's exclamation of surprise, the patient went on to say, "My dad shot me in the head. That's why my mom shot him dead." He explained, "My dad molested me until I was 17 years old." As the shocked chaplain tried to gather his thoughts and manage his feelings, the patient went on to share that the abuse began when he was 12. When his mother found out, she told the father to stop. "That's when he shot me." This happened 15 years ago.

Suddenly the patient asked the chaplain, "Would you do me a favor?" and without pausing went on to tell him his mother's nickname for him: "Squeaks," because of the way he cried. The patient then *asked the chaplain to hold him*, at which point he *broke into deep sobs*, mumbling something about a tape recorder to capture the "squeaks."

Description of what the practitioner, upon reflection,
considers most appropriate:

In what began as an ordinary visit to assess spiritual needs and provide spiritual care, the chaplain was starkly met with acute grief precipitated by the recent suicide of the patient's mother, and was taken aback by the grisly and complex nature of the patient's personal history. He would have been better prepared to respond to the patient's overwhelming need to be comforted had he conferred with other staff and read the patient's chart prior to the visit. In any case, the chaplain should have been careful to do so after the visit, reporting his findings and interaction in the patient's chart and in person to other treatment team members.

Background information that the practitioner considers useful:

John W. James and Russell Friedman, *The Grief Recovery Handbook*. New York: HarperPerennial, 1998.

Despair

Description of the client's circumstances
and the spiritual care offered:

The 80-year-old female patient with ovarian cancer, who was a self-identified Christian, *sought to share* with the chaplain her despair because of the length of her illness. Her energy level was low. Her two-month-long illness had made her "lose contact" with family, as she described it. When the chaplain asked what God meant to her, she said, "God is a companion to me in life. He is always with me." The chaplain then asked, "What about now? Where is God?" She replied, "Even in my sickness God is there. His will for me is more important." At that point, the chaplain did not seem to have anything more to say, so he offered a prayer and left.

Description of what the practitioner, upon reflection,
considers most appropriate:

The chaplain seemed to be asking formula-type questions to which the patient responded with textbook-type answers, leading to an impasse. Active listening coupled with empathetic and feeling responses would likely have enabled the patient to release some of her own anger, frustration, and sadness at her plight. At that point, the chaplain could have asked for her to share more of the story behind her loss of contact with loved ones. A life review could have been elicited in which the chaplain could affirm the patient's contributions to her family members. A closing prayer could have then included specifics meaningful to the patient.

Background information that the practitioner considers useful:

Erik H. Erikson, "Ego Integrity vs. Despair," *Childhood and Society*. New
York: Norton, 1963. 268–269.

Despair over Multiple Losses

Description of the client's circumstances
and the spiritual care offered:

The female Lutheran patient had been in a nursing/rehabilita-
tion facility for three years following the failure of her kidneys.
Other issues included diabetes, congestive heart failure, loss of
home, loss of job and financial independence, separation from
her daughter's life, and a sense of weakening faith. She was still
relatively young, but due to her circumstances she questioned
whether her future could be positive. Spiritual care needs were
related to allowing her to express her sense of weakening faith,
and to helping her reconnect to her faith community.

The chaplain had visited her often. On this occasion when he
asked how she was, she shared that she had just had a surprising
weight gain. This led to a *recounting of her story*, including many
serious difficulties with an abusive husband, a controlling mother,
and a teenage daughter with physical and developmental issues.
At one point, the patient *questioned the saying* that "God never
gives us more than we can handle," and *wept uncontrollably*. The
chaplain offered supportive responses throughout the visit and
concluded with a prayer.

Description of what the practitioner, upon reflection,
considers most appropriate:

If the chaplain could do this visit over, he would focus more on
inviting the resident to go deeper into her sense of God's abandonment and her image of God, perhaps leading to growth in
her understanding of God's presence and grace toward her in this
time of trial. The chaplain also could have helped the resident
open up more in the area of the cliché that "God never gives us

more than we can handle," which, while sounding pious, seldom attunes to the feelings of those who suffer.

Background information that the practitioner considers useful:

Erik H. Erikson, "Generativity vs. Stagnation." *Childhood and Society.* New York: Norton, 1963. 266–268.

Felicity Kelcourse, *Human Development and Faith: Life-Cycle Stages of Body, Mind, and Soul.* St. Louis: Chalice, 2004. 255–256.

Glendon Moriarty, *Pastoral Care of Depression: Helping Clients Heal Their Relationship with God.* Binghamton, NY: Haworth, 2006. 59–71.

Paul Tillich, *The Courage to Be.* New Haven: Yale University Press, 1952.

Despairing New Mother

Description of the client's circumstances and the spiritual care offered:

A 41-year-old female patient was tearful over many things, including a rejection of their new baby by the father and a lack of support by her friends. One friend had stayed with her during labor but then left. The patient had no connections with parents or siblings. She anticipated leaving the hospital the next day while her baby stayed to get nutrition via NG tube.

In this second visit, the chaplain was surprised by the amount of *sadness expressed* by the patient, since she had been fairly composed the day before. She offered reflective listening as the patient talked about many things, *crying* throughout the 20-minute visit.

The patient seemed to "give" the chaplain her problems to be solved, unable to see how she had contributed to her problems or how she could be a responsible mother. The chaplain encouraged the patient to (1) talk to her doctor regarding possible postpartum depression, and (2) hold her baby to help her focus on the love she felt for her. However, the patient seemed unable to engage these ideas as potential resources.

With the patient's *okay*, the chaplain prayed, touching the patient's shoulder with one hand and the baby with the other while the patient rested her hand on the baby: "Dear God, this is such a confusing time for (Patient). She loves (Baby) and is sad that she isn't eating well. Please send your healing power into (Baby)'s body and help her to keep growing. Comfort (Patient) that she is doing the best she can and that you are holding her in your arms right now. Give her peace that you will take care of her today and in the days ahead. You can be (Patient)'s husband, just as you are our Father and Mother. Send people to her that will care for her. We ask for strength and patience. Thank you for being with us. In your name we pray. Amen." The chaplain left with the patient's *thanks*.

Description of what the practitioner, upon reflection, considers most appropriate:

Ideally, the chaplain would have recognized earlier that the patient was too emotionally volatile to be able to engage in problem-solving. Should such a situation arise in the future, the chaplain would be more realistic about how much intervention can take place, provide a brief listening presence, and return later to follow up with more practical assistance.

The chaplain would also refrain from the use of medical terminology such as postpartum depression when speaking with the patient or staff. Instead, the chaplain would speak in spiritual assessment terms such as "despairing" or "deeply sad without a sense of resources or hope."

Background information that the practitioner considers useful:

Teresa Snorton and Jeanne Stevenson-Moessner, eds., *Women Out of Order: Risking Change and Creating Care in a Multicultural World.* Minneapolis: Fortress, 2010.

Despairing Shift from Caregiver to Care Receiver

Description of the client's circumstances
and the spiritual care offered:

A nurse paged the chaplain to the coronary care unit to attend to an elderly female patient who was feeling "down and depressed." The patient had just been given a long list of discharge orders (medication changes and exercise routines) to follow at home. The chaplain entered the room to find the patient propped up on the bed with IV lines running from her left arm and a nasal line on her face. The middle-aged son and daughter-in-law were sitting near the foot of the bed, the son engaged in a cell phone conversation. The patient had her head leaning back on the pillow with her eyes shut, moaning quietly.

The chaplain found herself with a woman in pain and dealing with the end of her life—not actually in a dying stage, yet still facing the end of healthy living. The chaplain tried to tap into her own memories of despairing feelings to help her reach out to the patient. She felt it would be healing to remind the patient of God's enduring presence, as a way to offer peace and comfort despite the frustrations of changes in routines and lifestyle.

As the conversation progressed, the patient said, "Yeah, been right with God a long time. Go to church when I can, but not lately 'cause of my legs. We got a new preacher there and I don't know him well. Nice enough young man, but he's not like our old one. He was there 40 years. I miss him. He gave powerful prayers." The chaplain responded, "You need powerful prayer right now? You know God wants to hear what's on your heart—willing to listen anytime. All you have to do is speak up."

The patient replied, "I know, I know. Been doing a lot of that today. Just don't feel like it's doing any good. I still feel low; just want to quit all this stuff. I'm in a real low place. So low I can't see up."

"May I try to pray for you?" the chaplain asked. The patient agreed. "*I'd like that.* Any praying gotta help."

The chaplain then prayed a prayer in which she herself reported feeling "lost in the holy moment," at the conclusion of which the patient *thanked her* and *asked her to stay* until her pastor arrived. The chaplain did so.

Description of what the practitioner, upon reflection, considers most appropriate:

The patient was clearly stressed with the complexities of her illnesses and the treatments prescribed for her. It was the chaplain's perception that, like many of the patient's generation, the older woman was used to being the caregiver for others and the source of strength within the family. Now she faced dependency upon others.

Also, the absence of her beloved pastor may have been part of her feeling an absence of God. It could have been helpful to invite her to speak more about this felt disconnection with God, perhaps with an open-ended question to her just after she said, "I'm in a real low place. So low I can't see up." For example, the chaplain could have asked, "When you pray to God, what do you say? What's on your mind and heart that you can share with God?"

Background information that the practitioner considers useful:

Joyce Rupp, *Praying Our Goodbyes*. Notre Dame, IN: Ave Maria, 1988.

Developmental Issues of a Critically Ill Teenager

Description of the client's circumstances and the spiritual care offered:

When the chaplain knocked on the door, the patient, a 16-year-old African American female, invited him into her room. He had been alerted to the patient's sickle cell disease by the chart and to her pain by the nurse. Having identified himself and gained her permission to enter, the chaplain asked if she would prefer to be alone. She said she would appreciate his visit and turned down the TV at his request as he took a seat near her bed.

After answering the chaplain's questions about her illness, she *moved the conversation to the humiliation* she was experiencing from her classmates and boyfriends in high school. With the chaplain's affirmation and support, she was able to describe her favorite school subject, her career dreams, and even her father's discouraging words about the possibilities for fulfilling those dreams. At that point, she became drowsy, having pressed the medication button early in the conversation according to her schedule. She fell asleep almost before the chaplain could close the conversation and wish her well.

Description of what the practitioner, upon reflection, considers most appropriate:

Though the patient's sickle cell illness caused her great physical pain, the emotional pain caused by those who humiliated her seemed equally great. In retrospect the conversation could perhaps have been more healing if the chaplain had been able to elicit more fully the patient's feelings of anger about her humiliation and her excitement about her dreams.

Background information that the practitioner considers useful:

Richard Dana, Lewis Bernstein, and Rosalyn S. Bernstein, *Interviewing: A Guide for Health Professionals*. New York: Appleton-Century Crofts, 1985.

Felicity Kelcourse, *Human Development and Faith: Life-Cycle Changes of Body, Mind, and Soul*. St. Louis: Chalice, 2004. 223.

Economic and Social Abandonment

Description of the client's circumstances and the spiritual care offered:

The chaplain encountered a husband and wife (each between 50 and 60 years of age) during the chaplain's afternoon rounding in the emergency department. Both individuals were in a corner of the waiting room, away from other patients and families, and appeared quiet.

The chaplain approached and inquired if they "felt cared for," to which the husband responded, "Not so much." This created a dialogue in which the couple—who showed consistency of thought and vision—expressed their economic hardship and related medical stress. The wife said, "Well, we just wait, you know? We know what's wrong; he just needs his medication. I *get tired* of the waiting—and the bills, my goodness, the bills. We don't make that kind of money, you know?"

The chaplain assessed for support and care contexts and discovered that the couple had previously been involved in community religious life through their Baptist church but no longer attended. ("We didn't really feel that connected to people," the wife said.) The chaplain identified with their struggle to create community by accessing his own faith heritage and history (also Baptist) with both a serious tone and appropriate use of humor. For instance, the Baptist chaplain apologized for a Baptist church that didn't work out and made a tongue-in-cheek promise of no business meetings during the visit. These jokes made the patients feel at ease, as evidenced by their *laughter*.

Prior to the husband's admission to the ER, the chaplain inquired if "creating church" through the ritual of prayer would be a helpful exercise of spirituality. Both individuals agreed and, after expressing their specific needs per the chaplain's inquiry, the chaplain prayed. "Lord, I thank you that we can create church here in this corner [*Husband:* Amen] and I thank you that we can struggle before you as a sympathetic God. [*Wife:* Yes] I pray for (Husband) and (Wife) as their day is long and trying, and for the physical healing that might take place through this hospital. I pray for the relief of stress that accompanies financial problems, and I join with them in that journey. [*Wife:* Yes] I ask for your provision, for your care, for your Spirit to be within them as they face this challenge together. And may you guide them toward others who can walk with them in our common faith. We ask these things in your name, amen." [*Husband and Wife:* Amen]

The visit concluded with the couple repeatedly *taking the chaplain's hand* while *expressing their gratitude* for his care.

Description of what the practitioner, upon reflection,
considers most appropriate:

Although the use of humor appeared appropriate and useful for defusing anxiety during an emergent medical situation, ideally the chaplain would have made a better assessment of the emotional state of the patient and family before introducing wit into the spiritual care context. Additionally the patient and family expressed a cycle of treatment through the use of emergency services that may have been best addressed through education by a member of the social work staff. A follow-up visit by the chaplain and a referral to the interdisciplinary staff may have assisted the patient and family in meeting their needs holistically.

Ectopic Pregnancy as Crushing News

Description of the client's circumstances
and the spiritual care offered:

A 30-year-old woman and her husband were in the middle of their second pregnancy. Their first pregnancy had ended with a miscarriage. The chaplain arrived just after doctors had told the couple this second pregnancy was an ectopic pregnancy and that there was no hope for the baby to be saved. The chaplain was paged by one of the ER nurses, who told him that the patient did not actually request a chaplain but was offered those services and was not opposed to the idea of a chaplain presence.

With her husband and brother present, and while grabbing at her side and wincing, the woman *tearfully shared* with the chaplain how she desperately wanted to become a mother and that she and her husband had been trying for "so long" to fulfill this dream. The chaplain expressed his sorrow at learning this. Several long, teary moments of silence followed. He checked with the husband, who responded matter-of-factly and without emotion that his first wife had also had an ectopic pregnancy. After more tearful silences and the chaplain's expressions of helplessness to do something, the woman *thanked* him for coming.

He then asked if she would like prayer. After a *yes*, he prayed: "God, life is painful sometimes. . . . We simply don't understand. Life hurts, but you promise to walk with us through the pain. Would you give (this couple) an extra sense of your presence? Would you wrap your arms around them and simply . . . hug them? As the doctors and the medical staff do what they need to do, would you work through them for the best possible outcome? Amen." Quickly turning to the husband to conceal his own tears, the chaplain let them know he was available for any other needs they may have. The chaplain made his exit.

Description of what the practitioner, upon reflection, considers most appropriate:

In terms of spiritual care, the chaplain believed the couple needed someone who was willing to listen and share the couple's burden. He also thought it was important for the woman to see that someone other than herself or her immediate family cared for this life that they loved and had been expecting to joyously bring into the world.

The chaplain believed that the moments of "holy silence" were healing. Upon reflection, the chaplain would not have shifted away from the woman's expressions of desperately wanting children to bring the husband into the conversation. Also, after the prayer the chaplain felt he should not have been afraid to look the woman in the eye despite his own tears. He concluded, "Looking her in the eyes, tears or no tears, just may have confirmed that God (whom I represented in this situation) cares for us when we suffer."

Background information that the practitioner considers useful:

Stanley Hauerwas, *God, Medicine, and Suffering.* Grand Rapids: Eerdmans, 1990.

Extreme Sense of Loss

Description of the client's circumstances and the spiritual care offered:

The patient was a 46-year-old male with a relatively youthful appearance who was a nominal Christian. The nurse indicated that he had a severe infection in his lower extremities and that no family members were identified as potential caregivers. The patient was sitting quietly in his bed at the far end of the hallway from the nurse's station, with the head of the bed at a slightly inclined angle. He had no one present with him. He was clean-shaven and had very few articles on his bedside table.

He was friendly in greeting the chaplain, expressing that he welcomed a visit. He spoke in a soft but intense voice when speaking of his mother ("Mommy") and of his physical suffering with his illnesses. There were no interactions with other staff or friends and family during the visit. In the initial phase of the visit, the patient *talked extensively* of the death of his mother two years prior and how he had cared for her at the expense of his own health. He spoke of the loss of his occupation as a cook and how much he had loved that occupation. He was currently on disability because of his continuing physical issues.

In describing his physical condition, he stated: "If you pointed a gun at me and told me to crawl over to that wall there or you would shoot me, I would tell you to just go ahead and get it over with. I just couldn't do it [make it over to the wall on his own power]." In a statement that reflected his hurt over his physical condition (in relationship to deity), he said, "You know, people do drugs, kill people, rape, steal, drink. I don't do any of that. And I do wonder . . . I don't even smoke. But I *wonder, 'Why?'*"

The chaplain responded with empathy, suggesting that characters in the Bible wondered that also and told God so. The chaplain then said, "It kind of sounds like you feel God has let you down. I think God understands that feeling." The patient said, "Yes, I know he does." When the chaplain asked if he could do anything for the patient, the man *requested prayer*. The chaplain asked if he had a specific request and the patient answered, "No, just pray."

The chaplain prayed, "Lord, I thank you for the courage that (Patient) has expressed, that he can keep going on. I pray that you will be with him and that he will find people who will stand by him. I pray in your name, amen." The patient said, "*Thank you so much.*" In parting, the chaplain said, "You are welcome," and left his card.

Description of what the practitioner, upon reflection, considers most appropriate:

The chaplain had scheduled this as the last visit of the day before needing to leave for a conference, and thus was aware it needed to be completed somewhat quickly. That element impacted the chaplain's ability to "stay with" the patient. The chaplain also admitted to having a certain emotional and mental psyche that "roots for the underdog." Further, he considered visiting the sick, the disadvantaged, and those in prison to be part of a personal theological mandate.

Upon reflection, it appeared the chaplain tended to be functioning more as a detective than as a chaplain during this visit. Although the chaplain gave the patient an outlet for his profound frustrations arising from his loss of health, family, and vocation, at several junctures it would have been beneficial to "stay with" the patient for a longer period of time as the visit progressed. Such junctures included when the patient spoke with deep emotion about the loss of his "Mommy" and how that had impacted him; when he expressed a deep hatred for his physical infirmities as he described his inability to move across the room even at gunpoint; and when he talked about the sinful or immoral acts others commit yet seemingly get away with, while bad things have happened to him. In all this, the patient felt he couldn't question God with "Why?" Each of those issues were ripe for deeper exploration.

Finally, the patient had asked for prayer. It would have been beneficial if the chaplain had delved into the patient's concept of

God, church affiliation, and other spiritual matters before venturing into prayer.

Background information that the practitioner considers useful:

Stephen B. Roberts, ed., *Professional Spiritual and Pastoral Care.* Woodstock, VT: SkyLight Paths, 2012.

Facilitating Staff Grief and Response to a Difficult Family Member

Description of the client's circumstances
and the spiritual care offered:

The kindly patient had been in hospice and had also received palliative care during her hospital stay. The patient, family, and patient's boyfriend were being supported by a cancer support services team.

The chaplain was called by the charge nurse to provide spiritual care to the family and the nursing staff after the patient's death, as well as to bring a peaceful presence, because while the family as a whole had been accepting of her impending death, one individual was not. At one point, the angry family member had begun yelling at God. The hospice representative intervened, stating it was okay to feel as he did. At that point, the man demanded all staff to leave the room. This left the nurses afraid of what might happen when the unaccepting person returned to view the body.

The chaplain initiated a brief defusing conversation, which provided the nurses an opportunity to *voice their fears, anxiety, and anger* about how the family member had treated them. The chaplain also facilitated collaborative dialogue among the care teams to assess and determine roles and to structure supportive care. The chaplain also represented the palliative care chaplain, per that colleague's request.

The hospice representative had been working with the daughters and thus supported them at the bedside when they arrived. The cancer support services team representative had also worked with everyone. He expressed that a chaplain's presence was most needed when working with angry individuals after a death.

Description of what the practitioner, upon reflection, considers most appropriate:

The chaplain was able to facilitate collaborative dialogue among the nurses, hospice, palliative care, and cancer support services teams in order to provide the family with supportive care following the death of a family member. The chaplain also provided defusing for the nurses prior to the family arriving to view the body, lowering their anxiety.

Outside the room, the chaplain could have coached the hospice representative about the spirituality of lament being expressed. The family member was crying out to God, who had just denied him his only request. Emotions were driving his words, so the best intervention was listening. The chaplain could have informed the hospice representative that the chaplain was listening to the family member and was okay with hearing harsh words toward God cried out during lament and grief. The chaplain could have listened more fully to the hospice representative and the nurse to honor the time they shared with the patient. This could have affirmed their spirituality of reminiscing and more appropriately validated their loss and grief for a patient they came to know and love for her kindness.

Background information that the practitioner considers useful:

William G. Dyer, W. Gibb Dyer Jr., and Jeffrey H. Dyer, *Team Building: Proven Strategies for Improving Team Performance,* 4th ed. Hoboken, NJ: John Wiley & Sons, 2010.

Paul F. Schmidt, *Coping with Difficult People.* Philadelphia: Westminster, 1980.

Fear of Cancer Recurrence

Description of the client's circumstances and the spiritual care offered:

The chaplain visited a 65-year-old female patient while on rounds at a rehab center. The patient asked the chaplain if he inspired hope in people. The patient also asked the chaplain if he prayed for people's cancer not to return. She shared that she had had a total of four surgeries because of her cancer, and that she did not want to talk about the cancer because she did not want it to return. She also shared that she wanted to postpone prayer for three days so her family could be present. The patient *shared excitement* when mentioning her family members but became silent after mentioning the son she had lost to an early death.

The chaplain tried to respect the patient's wish of not wanting to talk about the cancer and focused on the patient's family.

Description of what the practitioner, upon reflection, considers most appropriate:

Ideally, the chaplain would have joined the patient in her fear of the cancer returning, would have used "I" statements when discussing his own spiritual care giving, and would have sought to elicit more on her struggle with hope. Also, an invitation to further process her grief about her son's death could have been offered, such as, "I noticed that you grew silent at the mention of your son, and I felt sad." Finally, the chaplain would have invited the patient to prayer both at the present moment *and* later with the family.

Background information that the practitioner considers useful:

Resources from the Mayo Clinic and the American Cancer Society.
Gail Sheehy, *Passages*. New York: Ballantine, 1976.
Websites: www.cancer.org, www.cancercare.org,
     www.cancercareconnection.org

Feelings of Guilt and Disconnection, with Suicidal Ideation

Description of the client's circumstances
and the spiritual care offered:

A 16-year-old girl was admitted to the behavioral health unit because she was struggling to cope with feelings of betrayal and responsibility regarding family system issues. She became overstressed with the sudden changes in her life and, not knowing how to cope, attempted suicide by an overdose of ibuprofen.

This patient was in need of spiritual care in several areas. Upon discussion with the chaplain, *the story came to a fuller light*. This girl was left in charge of two younger siblings (ages 13 and 11), as her mother was the household income earner and had a job that lasted all night and into the late morning hours. With the mother absent overnight, the father had also been leaving and going a few blocks away to sleep with other women, unbeknownst to the mother or the children. One morning the girls missed the school bus and walked to an aunt's home. The patient, upon seeing her dad's truck outside, walked around back and let herself in the back door. She then discovered her dad in bed with another woman. The patient exited the house quietly (believing she had not been seen) and called her mother, who threw a fit, called for a divorce, and had since moved the children out of state with her. The patient told the chaplain that she believed her father was wrong, but she still loved him and missed him.

The patient *also shared* that she felt responsible for her parents' breakup, because she believed it was her phone call that brought the action into the light, causing her mother to break off the marriage. When the chaplain said, "You know it's not your fault, right?" she countered, "Yeah, I've been told and I guess I know it, but it's still hard."

The move required the patient to deal with making friends at a new school and adjusting to a new house, city, and state. The chaplain, identifying the girl's lack of connection to a support system, asked where she might find some healthy networks of support. The topic of church youth groups surfaced, and the girl remembered with fondness a time in the past when such a dynamic had existed in her life. The chaplain encouraged her to find out what possibilities existed in her area.

Through the course of the discussion, the patient mentioned that she felt she did not have anyone to share the load of life with, and that was when it became overwhelming. Thus, she thought it would be easier to end it all. Perceiving that the girl had nothing more to say, the chaplain concluded by asking if she would like a Bible. The patient answered with *an enthusiastic affirmative*; the chaplain left after saying he would be bringing her a Bible shortly and would be praying for her.

Description of what the practitioner, upon reflection, considers most appropriate:

The chaplain believed he had done some effective ministry but at the same time had missed some verbal cues to journey further with this patient's hurt and pain. He could have gone deeper in the discussion of how her father's betrayal made the patient feel. He could have asked if the family had been affected in any other emotional way, in addition to the obvious grief over the separation. When the patient had said, "It's still hard," the chaplain could have explored how it was hard for her. Finally, the chaplain could have gone one step further than simply encouraging her to seek social connection. He could have checked with churches in the area to find out if they provided transportation. (The patient had mentioned that she felt that connection would help yet worried that her mother would not support her in this area.)

Background information that the practitioner considers useful:

S. F. Shoemaker, "Adolescents," *Dictionary of Pastoral Care and Counseling.* Nashville: Abingdon, 1990. 8–10.

Feelings of Guilt and Shame

Description of the client's circumstances
and the spiritual care offered:

The patient was a Caucasian female in her seventies who was very thin, almost frail. She had undergone three surgeries as well as treatments for cancer, resulting in remission. This hospital admission had been for pneumonia. She had taken care of her chronically ill husband for a decade until his death the previous year. The patient expressed guilt about not supporting suggested treatment for her husband's bone cancer due to his dialysis, diabetes, and generally poor health. She noted conflict with in-laws, who blamed her for her husband's lack of treatment for this terminal illness and called her coldhearted for her inability to cry at the funeral. She also had deep issues around low self-esteem, feelings of unworthiness, and doubts about her own salvation. Furthermore, she was plagued by "what-ifs": What if he had received chemotherapy? What if he had been treated aggressively for his bone cancer? Was the doctor truly right in his assessment that the treatment would kill him? And so forth.

After introducing himself, the chaplain asked, "How's it going?" The patient *immediately went into her story* and her concerns. The chaplain said just the right words of encouragement and concern to enable her to share in depth and even *shed some of those long pent-up tears.* The chaplain's own self-revelation made it possible for her to say, "I have a lot of guilt. I keep praying, 'Jesus, don't leave me.'"

After more sharing, the chaplain asked and *got permission to pray.* Her choices for the prayer were for her health, that God would take her, and that the Lord would look after her daughters. The prayer was offered: "Dear Jesus, I pray for (Patient). I pray that your Spirit would comfort her. I pray, Lord, that you would give her strength and perseverance. Dearest Lord, please help her rest in your presence. Let her experience your acceptance in this room. I pray for her daughters, that you would give them peace and that you would comfort them about the terrible loss of their father. Lord, reassure (Patient) that she was a loving, caring wife. Help her to mourn her loss. Begin the healing of her body and spirit today. I ask these things in your name, Jesus. Amen."

The chaplain exited with the patient's *expressions of gratitude* for the visit.

Description of what the practitioner, upon reflection, considers most appropriate:

In retrospect the chaplain cited five indicators of success: (1) the patient's thoughts were turned to God and the patient was more conscious of God; (2) the patient, through the chaplain's visit, felt God's care, love, and active interest in her life; (3) the patient shared her burdens, including health issues, emotional pain, and hurts from the past, confessing things that had caused guilt, regret, and shame; (4) the patient entered into prayer with God; and (5) the patient felt glad that the chaplain had visited her.

Finding Meaning after Significant Losses

Description of the client's circumstances and the spiritual care offered:

During interdisciplinary morning rounds, the healthcare team noted that a post-surgery cardiac patient was depressed. When the chaplain visited, this patient told him that he was very tired, felt helpless and overwhelmed, and wasn't sure if he wanted to go on. The patient became teary as he *shared* that his wife had been killed in an automobile accident 10 years ago when a semitrailer truck sideswiped their car. His wife had died instantly, and he had suffered permanent injuries. In recounting these events, he said, "I just don't know why I am still here." (The patient had grown up in the Catholic faith but had became Protestant for the sake of his wife.) The chaplain prayed with the patient, who *expressed gratitude* for being able to share what was on his mind and heart. At the conclusion of the visit, the patient *appeared calmer.*

Description of what the practitioner, upon reflection,
considers most appropriate:

Ideally, the chaplain would have tried to elicit more about the patient's statement, "I just don't know why I'm still here." The chaplain could have invited the patient to take a walk around the unit. Along the way he could have asked more about his life and could have offered to arrange a visit from the clergy of his choice—Protestant or Catholic—or from a Eucharistic minister.

Background information that the practitioner considers useful:

James Brandis, "Why Am I Still Here? A Long-Term Chaplain Ponders."
   PlainViews 7:11, July 7, 2010.

Finding No Meaning in Life and Wanting to Die

Description of the client's circumstances
and spiritual care offered:

The chaplain, on rounds, visited a 90-year-old female patient who was brought to the ER with complaints of shortness of breath due to fluid in her lungs as a result of congestive heart failure. Upon entering the patient's room, the chaplain joked with the patient to establish a connection. (The elderly patient told him that he looked very young, and he told her the same!) The patient then revealed that she was raised in the Russian Orthodox Church, but that she was *having doubts* about believing in God due to the existence of suffering and death in the world. The patient expressed that she was not an atheist, but that she did not believe in God according to Christian thinking. She *stated that she wanted to die* because of her advanced age and, more importantly, because she could not find any meaning in her life. The patient also confided that she was tired of seeing other residents in her nursing home die.

The patient *asked the chaplain to explain his views* about God. Hesitantly, he explained some basic Christian theology concerning God as the Holy Trinity. As he had anticipated, his explanation seemed to have little effect on the patient's attitude. After the attempt to explain God theologically, he affirmed the patient's statements about God, a meaningless life, and seeing others around her die by using statements such as "You see others die" and "Uh-hmm."

Description of what the practitioner, upon reflection, considers most appropriate:

Joking with the patient helped the chaplain establish a better connection to lead into discussion about the patient's thoughts and feelings. Explaining theology was not very helpful. The patient's question about God could have been reframed and redirected, with the chaplain asking that the patient tell him her views about God instead of the other way around.

In addition, the chaplain should have investigated the patient's feelings of meaninglessness. It would have been helpful had the chaplain been curious about how the patient reached a level of disconnection with God and with others. The answer might have come from asking the patient about a time when she had meaning in her life, or if she ever felt there was meaning in her life. Lastly, prayer may have been helpful to strengthen the patient's wavering faith.

Background information that the practitioner considers useful:

Erik H. Erikson, *Childhood and Society*. New York: Norton, 1963. 268–269.

Frustrated and Grieving Son of a Patient

Description of the client's circumstances and the spiritual care offered:

While the chaplain was doing rounds in the ICU and conducting initial assessments, the unit RN told her that a 75-year-old Vietnamese American female with stage IV cancer was unresponsive, but that the patient's son, described as "very emotional" and having no support, might benefit from a visit despite the fact that they didn't "go to church."

The chaplain found the son just outside his mother's room, identified herself, and responded to his request to find a place to sit since he was feeling weak. He then *readily and tearfully shared his story*: his dying mother was his best friend; his dilemma about burial arrangements, wanting to take her back to Vietnam but not being able to afford it; his sadness and anger at life; his singleness at age 49; his sleeplessness; and his desire for the chaplain to continue to check in on him and his mother.

The visit concluded with the son asking whether he could sleep there [*Editor's note:* actual location not reported] and the chaplain saying that he could do so. When she noted that other chaplains were available, he *stated his preference for only her*.

Description of what the practitioner, upon reflection, considers most appropriate:

The chaplain became determined to conduct this visit—after hearing that the patient's son may not need a chaplain because they were not Christians—in part as a learning for the RN that chaplains stand alongside all persons in connecting with the joy and pain that patients go through, irrespective of personal beliefs or worldviews.

The chaplain used the spiritual care approach of listening thoughtfully and openly without diverting to elements of the stories as the patient's son continued to share. Upon reflection, it could have been healing for the patient's son if the chaplain had invited him to the feeling level by saying things like, "What's it feel like to. . . ?" and to affirm him by saying, "I am glad I could keep you company for this time." On a practical note, she could have asked, "What's the best time to visit you again?"

Background information that the practitioner considers useful:

M. Scott Peck, *A World Waiting to Be Born: Civility Rediscovered*. New York: Bantam, 1993. 294.

Grief and Contrition in Loss of Contact with Daughter

Description of the client's circumstances and the spiritual care offered:

By the patient's account, she had been in a placement facility for at least four years prior to being admitted to the behavioral health unit the day before the chaplain's visit. At first resistive, the patient was later *moved to tears* by the chaplain's comment, "Your eyes look so sad!" After a hard cry of release, she described her loss of visiting privileges with her four-year-old daughter, who had been adopted last August in an "open adoption." The patient *expressed what she described as her selfishness* that led to that loss. Her repeated phrase "I was so selfish" seemed to *express genuine contrition* but also a sense of hopelessness and loss that she felt very deeply.

In a story punctuated with spells of crying and tears, the patient related how she had placed her daughter for adoption. She evidently had developed a good relationship with the adoptive parents and had been able to visit her daughter often. She related how the adoptive parents continued to help her keep in touch with her daughter and how they had been so nice to her. She stated the adoption "was working out okay."

According to her story, while continuing to live in the group home, she experienced difficulty sleeping. She received regular medication for "bipolar and other stuff" from staff at the group home. However, without the knowledge of staff, she found some sleep medication and was taking it so she could sleep better. The patient added, "They found out about it . . . and so I had to leave . . . and now I can't see my daughter because I was so selfish . . . and I don't even have a place to go to now."

The patient *asked for prayer* and then told the chaplain what he could pray for: "Pray for my daughter that she will be okay." He prayed, "Dear Lord, I pray for (Daughter), that you would comfort her. I pray that you would hold her in your arms and protect her and give her understanding. I pray for (Patient) as well, that you would bring comfort to her, that she can begin to get peace about this. Help her as she prepares for the future, that she would understand what it is that you have for her. And I pray that somehow it might work out someday for her to see her daughter again. Thank you. Amen."

The patient *thanked* him, and he closed the conversation with an affirmation of her courage.

Description of what the practitioner, upon reflection, considers most appropriate:

Upon reflection, the chaplain's sensitive observation ("Your eyes look so sad!") opened the patient to a healing catharsis as she released her tears and then shared her deep concerns and contrition. At the same time, there was a sense that the chaplain could have helped the patient more in her struggle with the painful consequences of her perceived selfishness. In response to the patient's self-condemnation of selfishness, the chaplain might have said, "Help me to understand the feelings you have concerning what you feel was selfish in your actions." In response to the patient's despair over her choices and consequences, the chaplain might have said, "You speak of such a strong feeling of pain and hopelessness. Could you help me to understand what that is like for you?" (In this response, the chaplain would be attempting to explore with the patient what it is really like to be in her situation, or entering the patient's frame of reference.) Finally, before praying, it would have been wise for the chaplain to explore what "okay" would have looked like for the patient. That is, the chaplain could have sought to help her articulate her hope for a better—but realistic—future for her daughter.

Background information that the practitioner considers useful:

Stephen B. Roberts, ed., *Professional Spiritual and Pastoral Care: A Practical Clergy and Chaplain's Handbook.* Woodstock, VT: SkyLight Paths, 2012.
Froma Walsh and Monica McGoldrick, eds., *Living Beyond Loss.* New York: Norton, 1991.

Grief at the Death of a Young Mother

Description of the client's circumstances and the spiritual care offered:

The chaplain "walked" with an older sister and the seven-year-old son of a comatose patient on an end-of-life "journey" that lasted four days. During that journey, they *talked of good-byes* and the chaplain helped the boy say good-bye to his mother. The sister talked with the chaplain about her process of obtaining guardianship of her nephew. She *reflected on the life of the patient*, which included all of her "should-haves." Lastly, they *discussed the patient's code status*, including the sister's inevitable decision, as the healthcare surrogate, and the withdrawal of all life support.

The sister was *transparent with her emotions and anxieties* about losing her sister. She was tearful as she related all of her losses (both parents, two siblings, and two cousins within the past three years) and now this unexpected crisis with her baby sister. She *related her grief* for her nephew and the responsibilities of raising him that now would be hers. She *questioned* how she should talk to him about his mother. The chaplain shared her sense that children are quite resilient, and that often they can see the reality of a situation better than adults can. The chaplain was able to speak with the patient's son outside the room and then assisted him in saying good-bye, in his way, to his mother at her bedside.

Description of what the practitioner, upon reflection, considers most appropriate:

The chaplain offered herself and her caring in an open and non-judgmental way by valuing this sister and all of her losses and grief. The chaplain was frustrated afterward with not having resources about grief for both the sister and the son. Upon reflection, the following approaches were seen as ideal: (1) caring for each person in an open and nonjudgmental way; (2) listening to the sister's lament and being present to her during the code status talk; (3) listening to the son's lament; and (4) following up with a sympathy card and a packet containing grief resources for reading, grief support groups for both adults and children, and parenting tips.

Background information that the practitioner considers useful:

Kenneth R. Mitchell and Herbert Anderson, *All Our Losses, All Our Griefs.* Louisville: Westminster John Knox, 1983.

Alan D. Wolfelt, *Healing a Child's Grieving Heart: 100 Practical Ideas for Families, Friends and Caregivers.* Ft. Collins, CO: Companion, 2001.

Grief Ministry with a Fellow Passenger

Description of the client's circumstances
and the spiritual care offered:

While flying to a conference, the chaplain entered into conversation with her seatmate. The woman was on her way to help care for a sick aunt. Her own mother had died just four months earlier. As the chaplain listened, the passenger *recounted her last days with her mother*, shedding *a few tears* in the process. The chaplain "validated her tears," giving acknowledgment in the form of "verbal listening."

The chaplain also asked a few leading questions (for instance, "How are you coping?"), which her fellow passenger answered "with reservations." However, during the conversation the chaplain thought it somewhat strange that her fellow passenger was so open so quickly.

Description of what the practitioner, upon reflection,
considers most appropriate:

In retrospect the chaplain felt that her effort was effective: the woman needed to share her story and the chaplain allowed her to do so. The chaplain later summarized, "I'm not sure that I would do anything differently. . . . We were in an unusual place with limited time."

Perhaps the passenger's readiness to share was enhanced by a sense of her listener's special sensitivity; the chaplain's own mother had died just one year before.

Grieving and Distressed Staff

Description of the client's circumstances and the spiritual care offered:

The chaplain was walking toward her office when she saw another staff member in the hallway and said hello. The staff member responded, "Hey, there's my friend!" The chaplain asked how she was doing. The staff member *shared* that her family had just lost a cousin and that she and her husband were taking care of the deceased's children. The staff member went on to state that it was difficult seeing the pain and grief that the children were experiencing, especially the 13-year-old daughter. She also shared that they were also dealing with a flooded basement, and that her husband had been pulled over for speeding with children in the back who weren't in car seats. The result of the ticket was to pay out money they didn't have at the time.

The chaplain provided a listening ear, empathic responses, and a comforting presence. The staff member's *affect noticeably brightened* as she was enabled to tell her story. In parting, the chaplain said, "See you later, and when you need to talk to someone, you know where to find me."

Description of what the practitioner, upon reflection, considers most appropriate:

The importance of an ongoing and supportive general presence in the hospital was highlighted in the staff member's greeting to the chaplain. Rapport was already clearly established, making it easier for the staff member to share her troubling story.

In retrospect the chaplain noted that she had been able to inwardly draw upon her own grief experience, thereby authenticating her empathic responses. She rightly felt that the most appropriate and potentially effective spiritual care intervention for this person was the service provided.

Ideally, the chaplain would have arranged a follow-up meeting, perhaps for coffee, with the staff member before parting so that more care could be provided. Given no mutual follow-up arrangements made on the spot, the chaplain could have taken the initiative a few days later to discreetly seek out the staff member to see how she was faring.

Background information that the practitioner considers useful:

Pamela Cooper-White, *Shared Wisdom: Use of Self in Pastoral Care and Counseling.* Minneapolis: Fortress, 2004.

Grieving Patient as "Difficult Patient"

Description of the client's circumstances
and the spiritual care offered:

Nursing staff called the chaplain to visit a patient who was considered "difficult." Upon arriving on the floor, the chaplain was notified that the patient's mother had died the previous day. The chaplain entered the patient's room and introduced himself. The patient appeared angry and was attempting to get out of bed to plug in his cell phone. While helping the patient plug in the phone, the chaplain asked if the cell phone's battery was dead. The patient responded that things had been dying all his life. After the patient's statement, the chaplain laughed at this description of death in his life related to the battery's death. However, the patient became very angry, yelled, and used foul language. During the course of the visit, the chaplain listened to the patient's *story of grief* related to his mother's death, his own health problems (including hepatitis C), and his concerns and anger toward his family and the people he believed were taking advantage of them.

Along with this story, the patient spoke about getting more closely connected with his church and with God. He *expressed disappointment* with this relationship. During the patient's story, the chaplain did not meet the patient's intensity. As the patient yelled, the chaplain tried to respond in ways that would calm the patient. The chaplain also did not respond to the patient's disappointment about not being able to be part of the planning of his mother's funeral because of his own health and lack of finances. Also, when the patient threatened to cause harm to those who interfered with his family, the chaplain began to judge the patient.

Description of what the practitioner, upon reflection, considers most appropriate:

Ideally, the chaplain would have been more perceptive about the patient's hurt and grief. Instead of laughing at the patient's metaphorical statement relating the death of his cell phone battery to death in his own life's experiences, the chaplain would have noticed that the patient was grieving.

Next, the chaplain would have met the patient's powerful, angry statements and yelling with more responsive and intense statements instead of immediately trying to calm the patient. Further, he would have heard more carefully the patient's disappointment, anger, and grief related to being excluded from planning his mother's funeral as a result of his own health struggles. He would have noticed that the patient's threats to harm others were related to his own helplessness and desire to feel powerful during a critical time in his life.

The chaplain might have focused more on the patient's relationship with God and the disappointment he felt in himself as related to this relationship. Furthermore, the chaplain could have engaged the patient on his statements concerning his experience in church life and explored the meaning of these life-giving experiences. Before ending the visit, it would have been helpful to offer prayer at the patient's bedside.

Background information that the practitioner considers useful:

C. Charles Bachmann, *Ministering to the Grief Sufferer.* Englewood Cliffs, NJ: Prentice-Hall, 1964.

Guilt about Not Being Present at the Death of a Spouse

Description of the client's circumstances
and the spiritual care offered:

The chaplain arrived at work and learned that a patient had died 30 minutes earlier. The patient's wife had been called. Upon her arrival, the chaplain was notified and entered the room. In the first five minutes of the conversation, the deceased's wife asked three times, "Why did he have to die alone?"

The chaplain focused on the wife's misunderstanding that the patient was alone in the room when he died, and tried to assure her that other staff members had been present. The chaplain then realized that the wife was really asking why *she* was not there when her husband died. At that point, the chaplain was able to move from data to feelings and hear the wife's lament. The wife was then *able to share more* about times in their marriage when they had been separated and how she had navigated those times.

Description of what the practitioner, upon reflection,
considers most appropriate:

Ideally, the chaplain would not have interpreted the wife's question so literally and would have more carefully listened for what might have been behind the words. When the wife asked, "Why did he have to die alone?" the chaplain could have said something like, "I might be asking, 'Why did he have to die *without me there beside him?*'" The wife might then have been more able to share her guilt about not having been with the patient at the moment of his death. The conversation could perhaps have moved more smoothly into times during their marriage when they had been separated from one another and each had felt alone. The chaplain could then have invited the wife to share ways in which she navigated those lonely times and also could have suggested bereavement resources available to her in the community, such as a local religious leader or hospice programs.

Background information that the practitioner considers useful:

Penelope Wilcock, *Spiritual Care of Dying and Bereaved People*. New York: Morehouse, 1997.

Impromptu Ministry in the Shock of Bad News

Description of the client's circumstances
and the spiritual care offered:

The chaplain was walking from a building adjoining the hospital into the patient entrance, deep in thought, and spoke a perfunctory but friendly greeting to a middle-aged man: "How are you today?" When the man replied, "Other than having been told that I have a brain tumor and it can't be operated on and there is no medicine to touch it, that I am going to die with it, I am okay," the chaplain was jolted out of his thoughts of the moment. When he realized the pain involved in the patient's response, he made an instantaneous commitment to join the man in conversation. They stood by the entrance as they continued conversing. People walked by as they conversed, but the man seemed oblivious to that as the conversation continued. The chaplain inquired whether the man wanted to move to a more private location, but he declined because he was waiting for a friend to come pick him up and was to be at the entrance.

The (assumed) patient was tall, quite unkempt in appearance, visibly agitated, and apparently in a situation where he felt the need to speak with someone about his dilemma. The chaplain judged him to be approximately 45 years old. He *spoke with intensity and considerable depth of feeling.* He was alone.

The patient's initial response became the focal point of the conversation. As the conversation unfolded, the patient revealed he had been initially diagnosed with an inoperable brain tumor at a VA hospital and had come in for a second opinion. He appeared stunned that this diagnosis was identical to what he had been told at the VA. He said he was a 15-year Army Ranger veteran who had fought in many battles and was going to fight this disease with the same urgency and courage, even though he knew it ultimately would kill him.

As the chaplain attempted to explore with the patient the support system he had to stand by him, the patient *revealed a further source of personal pain.* His wife was "fighting [him] all the way," not even letting him fully explain to their children what was happening to him. The patient was *able to identify a few supports* that he did have available to him as he entered this battle of and for his life, including his Catholic heritage. As the conversation ended, he *thanked* the chaplain for talking with him but declined an offer of prayer, saying, "Naw, I'm fine. Just say some prayers for me." The chaplain agreed, and they parted company.

Description of what the practitioner, upon reflection, considers most appropriate:

The chaplain did explore with the patient some of his initial feelings but could have stayed with him in his pain for a more extended time, focusing primarily on the shock and pain of the diagnosis. Included in this would also be further exploration of his perceived abandonment by his wife in this time of need and his feeling that he was also not supported by her in preparing their children for his ordeal.

By way of ongoing support, the chaplain helped the patient identify such things as talking to his priest and looking into participation in an existing support group through the VA hospital system. It would also have been helpful for the chaplain to honor the patient's notation of being part of a local Catholic parish by offering to facilitate contact with a priest of that parish.

Background information that the practitioner considers useful:

Stephen B. Roberts, ed., *Professional Spiritual and Pastoral Care: A Practical Clergy and Chaplain's Handbook.* Woodstock, VT: SkyLight Paths, 2012.

Lamenting Lost Motherhood

Description of the client's circumstances and the spiritual care offered:

While the patient was intubated in ICU for nearly a week following an operation to remove fluid from around her heart, the chaplain visited several times with her husband, her daughter, and her brother, who had donated a kidney to her 10 years earlier. The brother said the kidney had stopped functioning about 5 years earlier and that she needed a new transplant. The 36-year-old patient was in renal failure, and her husband said she had been "very sick" for 14 years.

About 24 hours after she was extubated, the chaplain visited the woman, still weak and only able to speak slowly and softly. The chaplain told the patient that she could stop the conversation if she became tired, but she *very much wanted to talk.* She shared about her illness in some detail, describing her pain as "crippling," and when the chaplain asked how she coped, she replied, "I pray like hell." This was a bit of a surprise to the chaplain because her family did not seem at all religious.

When asked what she prayed for, she *said she asked God* for enough time (about five months) to see their only child, an 18-year-old girl, graduate from high school. She then said she hoped God would give her enough time to see a grandchild. The patient *lamented,* "I never got to see my daughter grow up," and now she would not get to enjoy her grandchildren. She had cried several times and was getting weaker. The chaplain, realizing he must soon end the visit, asked if she could see God in her pain, hoping the long-praying patient could find hope in her fervent prayers. When she *confirmed a hope in God,* the chaplain responded to the patient's request for prayer for more time, and after prayer the visit ended.

Description of what the practitioner, upon reflection,
considers most appropriate:

The visit gave the patient space to explore the pain and loss surrounding her illness, and to reinforce her faith and hope by eliciting these words from her: "I keep praying—what else can I do?" The patient concluded that she could still experience God's love in her pain, and requested that the chaplain pray with her for more time, thus providing a strengthening of the patient's faith.

Upon reflection, the chaplain concluded that the exploration of the pain surrounding her illness could have been shorter. This could have allowed the patient to benefit more from lamenting in depth about the perceived unfairness of her illness, which she saw as robbing her of the ability to be an active participant in raising her only daughter.

The chaplain, realizing time was a factor, could have encouraged her mourning the loss of her motherhood more deeply, thereby adding to the value of the visit. The lament of lost motherhood was likely more important during this first visit than exploring the love of God in her illness, something better reserved for a second visit.

Background information that the practitioner considers useful:

Pamela D. Larsen and Irene Morof Lubkin, *Chronic Illness: Impact and Intervention*. Burlington, MA: Jones & Bartlett, 2009. 197.

Paul W. Powell and Arthur E. Dell, *Families Living with Chronic Illness and Disabilities*. Chicago: Ortho Atlas, 2004.

Loneliness

Description of the client's circumstances
and the spiritual care offered:

While on usual rounds in a cardiac unit, the chaplain encountered a female patient in her late twenties. She was lying in bed with the television on. The room was bare; no cards, flowers, or personal items were visible. It was a dark and gloomy day outside, so the only light in the room came from the light over the patient's bed, which added to the clinical feeling of the room. The patient's energy level seemed extremely low.

The chaplain introduced himself and explained spiritual care services. The patient invited him to visit with her for awhile. He took a chair next to the patient's bed and asked how she was doing. She explained her physical symptoms and her experience of fear from not being able to catch her breath. The patient had a perceived need to talk and to be heard, but the chaplain did not sense that she had a well-developed spiritual life. No church connection was indicated in her file. Her family consisted only of her mother, who lived with her. (An aunt had drifted apart from the family.) The patient was out of touch with old girlfriends. She did some hairdressing and nail work, and had thought about going to school for more formal training in cosmetology. Sensing some interest there, the chaplain encouraged her to pursue this schooling. He offered prayer, and the patient seemed grateful, *inviting him to come back* whenever he could.

The chaplain stopped by the next day, but the patient indicated she felt quite ill and was not up for conversation. She extended her arms, and they *hugged* good-bye. The next time the chaplain was on the unit, the patient had been released.

Description of what the practitioner, upon reflection, considers most appropriate:

The patient's immediate need seemed to be for company to alleviate feelings of loneliness and isolation, most likely heightened due to her illness and hospitalization. Questions could have been asked to determine her spiritual life, especially in light of her sense of loneliness. The best intervention with this patient would have been active listening, allowing her to lead the conversation yet picking up on the feelings behind the words.

Although the issue the chaplain presented to his colleagues was how to get out of a visit gracefully that is lasting too long or not accomplishing anything, his colleagues discerned that he was the one prolonging the conversation with a series of questions. Colleagues also saw the patient's loneliness and isolation, and expressed their opinion that the chaplain did not explore her feelings in the original visit and did not encourage her to talk about the sense of loneliness and depression she presented. More appropriate questions would have been "How did that make you feel?" and "When I hear you talk about your family, I hear some loneliness and sadness in your voice. Is that how you are feeling?" Regarding going to cosmetology school, the chaplain might have asked, "Is there something stopping you from doing that?"

Loneliness with Physical and Emotional Pain

Description of the client's circumstances and the spiritual care offered:

The patient, a 95-year-old female with chronic heart failure and pneumonia, had been in and out of the hospital several times in recent months. In previous visits with the chaplain, the patient did not refrain from expressing her feelings and sense of struggle. She had moved many miles away from her home area a few years earlier. She had five daughters living locally and one son "back home" whom she rarely saw. Each daughter had challenges, including one whose husband had committed suicide and another who was separated from her husband and child. When the chaplain previously commented that the patient had been through a lot of challenges lately, she had said, "I have suffered like none other."

At the time of this visit, the patient was nauseated and in discomfort. Nonetheless, as "an affectionate person," she *greeted the chaplain with warmth* on this occasion. He took her hand and stood by the head of her bed, eliciting stories about her children and her illness, and responding to her with emotional reflection (using words to reflect back, as a way to check and validate her feelings).

The patient responded well to sympathetic and empathetic listening. Near the end of the visit, the patient *asked the chaplain to pray.* He did so, praying for the above-mentioned concerns by name and for God's presence of peace and comfort for her while in the hospital. At the close of the prayer, the patient *expressed her gratitude.*

Description of what the practitioner, upon reflection, considers most appropriate:

The patient needed to tell someone outside the family unit about her family concerns. In many ways the patient was a very expressive person who respected clergy and needed a sensitive listening ear. Her expression of thanks at the conclusion of the visit validated the chaplain's success in providing much-needed healing care.

Long-Term Grief over Spouse's Unexpected Suicide

Description of the client's circumstances and the spiritual care offered:

The chaplain was making rounds at a rehab hospital and doing initial assessments. In one room, the male patient seemed to be asleep, so the chaplain quietly left her card on the meal tray and turned to leave. At that point, the patient spoke, giving her a friendly smile and asking her not to go.

When the patient learned that she was a chaplain, he identified himself as having attended the Church of the Brethren for 30 years. He had not returned there for the past eight years—ever since his wife, who suffered with Lou Gehrig's disease, had shot and killed herself one day without having ever given any sign of wanting to take such drastic action. The patient *shared his ongoing inability to understand* how and why that could have happened, especially since it was a total surprise to him. The chaplain responded with active listening and empathetic comments.

The patient *asked the chaplain* whether those who commit suicide go to hell. She answered that she personally did not believe so. The patient went on to describe his pastor's position—similar to that of the chaplain's—and what a helpful message his pastor had delivered at his wife's funeral. The chaplain followed with more empathetic comments.

The patient went on to *describe his health situation*, being in recovery from both a bout with cancer and knee surgery. The chaplain continued with empathetic listening and responses.

The conversation was interrupted by a telephone call that the patient chose to take—he had been anticipating this call from his "significant other"—and the chaplain took her leave.

Description of what the practitioner, upon reflection, considers most appropriate:

The chaplain provided a supportive and listening presence, allowing the patient to talk about his devastation at the abrupt loss of his wife to suicide as well as about his own health issues. The patient invited the chaplain to journey with him into that most difficult area—suicide—and she did so, albeit briefly.

In retrospect the patient would have been well served had she tried to elicit a deeper, more healing conversation about the patient's feelings toward suicide and about what his wife's loss continues to mean to him in "feeling" terms.

Background information that the practitioner considers useful:

Parker J. Palmer, *Let Your Life Speak: Listening for the Voice of Vocation.* San Francisco: Jossey-Bass, 2001.

Loss, Grief, and Guilt

Description of the client's circumstances and the spiritual care offered:

The chaplain conducted an initial assessment visit with an unmarried 28-year-old male patient on disability, having been unable to work since age 25 due to his illness. He had been admitted to a continuous critical progressive unit the day before with a collapsed lung and was being stabilized for surgery to remove a portion of his right lung the following week. During the visit, the patient *stated he blamed himself for his medical condition*, evidently feeling it had been brought on by his choices.

Intertwined in the story of his medical condition was a recurring narrative of his relationship with his paternal grandfather. He had gained a great deal of computer expertise from his grandfather, who apparently had been very successful in computer technology and had passed along this knowledge. The patient *lamented the loss* of his ability to earn a living due to his illness: "I *want* to work, I *love* to work, but I can't."

When asked about denominational or faith affiliation, the patient identified a local church that he sometimes attended. The patient also introduced the idea that his grandfather had been quite critical of some of the choices he had made regarding friends and of activities in which he had been involved. At one point, the patient spoke of his being with friends, only to have them steal and swindle from him, which led to his grandfather "yelling" at him. He *exhibited considerable anxiety* over his continuing dilemma concerning choices of friends and activities, stating often, "I just don't know what to do."

The patient's mother and her parents were initially present. Later in the visit, only the patient was present. As the conversation continued, the patient appeared quite nervous and upset but didn't seem to know how to speak openly about the nature of some of his illnesses, although overall he was quite articulate.

With the patient's *permission,* the chaplain concluded the visit with this prayer: "Dear Lord, you know (Patient) and the dilemma he finds himself in. I pray for your wisdom for him and that you would help him deal with these issues. I pray for your protection over him as he goes into surgery. Thank you for your wisdom you give so freely. Amen." The chaplain then departed with the patient's *thanks*.

Description of what the practitioner, upon reflection, considers most appropriate:

The chaplain did not explore why the patient felt his disease was his fault. The chaplain felt the patient was guarded about it and didn't seem to want to divulge information. However, the patient's seeming agitation about his illness and especially about his reported relationship with his grandfather left the chaplain somewhat frustrated in knowing how to respond. All indications were that the patient wanted to talk but didn't know what to say or how to say it. The visit also felt quite disjointed as the chaplain had to leave several times to allow nursing staff to make preparations for the patient's imminent discharge.

In retrospect it appeared that the patient was grieving the loss of his identity. A focus that became clear was the need to allow the patient to shape his own story. In such an exchange, the chaplain ideally would become the guide for the patient rather than the one establishing the course of the conversation. For example, when the patient said, "My medical problems began when I was 25. . . . I have had all kinds of things happening since then," the chaplain's response could have been to join with the patient by asking, "All kinds of things? What are those things?" When the patient identified a church experience, albeit a tenuous one, the chaplain could have asked, "What was that experience like?" or "Have you ever felt God's presence?" When the patient shared about his friends ripping him off and his grandfather yelling at him, the chaplain could have tried to validate the story and the feelings associated with it to help the patient feel understood. Finally, reading the patient's history and intentionally thinking of what the chaplain might feel in a similar situation could have helped. Follow-up with staff "in the loop" also would have been most helpful.

Background information that the practitioner considers useful:

Norman Cousins, *The Healing Heart: Antidotes to Panic and Helplessness.*
New York: Norton, 1983.

Loss of Personal Independence

Description of the client's circumstances
and the spiritual care offered:

The chaplain was doing a follow-up visit requested by the chaplain who had done the initial visit with this patient, a female Roman Catholic. She had a small brain bleed as well as macular degeneration in both eyes. She did not remember any injuries to her head.

It was already dark outside when the chaplain arrived at the patient's room. The patient was in the bed closest to the door, and the other bed was unoccupied. The room was dimly lit. The television was on, but the patient had her back to the TV. There were no cards, flowers, or other evidence of well-wishers, and her bedside table was empty. There were no IVs or monitors present in the room.

The patient's initial expressed concern was "Oh, I've been better." The patient mentioned her macular degeneration and then told the chaplain that she had blood in her brain that her doctor told her would take care of itself without medical intervention. As the conversation continued, she told him she lived alone and one of her sons would be coming to stay with her. At one point she said that life was dismal and then elaborated. She would need someone to live with her because of her deteriorating vision, but she was hesitant to ask any of her very busy adult children. Her *expressed hope* was that her right eye would improve as the blood in her brain dissipated. At that point, the chaplain was paged. He quickly determined her faith—Catholic—and that she would like Communion. He said he would arrange it, and she *expressed her thanks* for that. The chaplain offered a prayer before responding to the page.

Description of what the practitioner, upon reflection,
considers most appropriate:

The patient was able to share about her vision problems, her feeling that life would be dismal without her eyesight, and her dread
about needing help at home. The chaplain was able to make the
connections necessary so that she could receive Communion. She
expressed appreciation for that.

Given another opportunity, the chaplain could more intentionally stay with the underlying dynamics expressed by the patient—
feelings of grief, loss, loneliness, fear, and sadness—rather than
moving to a more positive statement of hope about her right eye.

Overwhelming Sense of Failure

Description of the client's circumstances
and the spiritual care offered:

The patient was a 70-year-old, married Baptist male suffering
from back pain, COPD, lung cancer, and shortness of breath. The
on-duty chaplain from the previous evening had spoken briefly
with the patient and indicated that he appeared to want to talk
more and might profit from a follow-up visit. In the follow-up
visit, the chaplain entered the room and found the patient asleep.
As the chaplain slipped his calling card onto the bedside stand,
the patient awoke and invited the chaplain to stay and visit. He
appeared somewhat unkempt and was unshaven. No one else
was present during the visit. A nurse's aide entered at one point to
take some routine measurements of blood pressure, temperature,
and the like.

As the conversation developed, it was apparent that the patient
had been doing some serious thinking and was quite anxious to
speak with a chaplain or someone else interested in helping him
with his spiritual dilemma. The patient was *very intense and serious* as he began the conversation and *became quite emotional* at
one point. His two opening statements set the tone for the visit as
he said, "I can never go back to where I once was. *I have made*

too *many mistakes*, failed too many times," and "I have been given so many opportunities, I have blown so many of them, I have made so many mistakes. . . . I don't know if I can ever get back to God. I don't know if it is possible."

The chaplain responded, "It sounds like you feel you have made so many mistakes that God could never accept you back." The patient agreed with that description. He then indicated that part of his dilemma was that he felt "getting back to God" involved attending church. He had gotten out of the pattern of going because his wife had been "hurt by church people" and refused to go with him. For him, however, the issue remained that he felt that he had failed God too many times to ever go back to the Lord again. The chaplain responded with reflective listening, a reference to the prodigal son story, appropriate self-revelation, and a note of hope ("The fact that you are so concerned about your relationship with God tells me you have not gone too far, that you are *not* unforgivable, unpardonable."). Finally, the chaplain responded willingly to the patient's request for prayer. The patient responded with "*Thanks*. That means a lot to me. Thanks so much." He also *stated a desire to try to return to church* with or without his wife, and *requested that the chaplain pay a return visit.*

Description of what the practitioner, upon reflection, considers most appropriate:

The chaplain sought to minister in terms of the grace and forgiveness of God. Early in the conversation, the chaplain responded well to the patient's opening remarks about not being able to get back to God and of having made too many mistakes with an active listening response, as affirmed when the patient agreed with his observation.

It would have been helpful if the chaplain had helped the patient explore his concept or view of God and how that impacted him. Exploration of his Baptist faith tradition, and how that had contributed to his sense of either God being unforgiving or his inability to return to God, would also have been helpful. Those avenues of inquiry might have revealed the reasons behind the patient's sense of failure. The chaplain's tendency in this conversation was to move too quickly to offering a patient a sense of hope. In so doing, the focus was turned away from helping the patient rediscover his own belief system so that he could use it as an empowering resource on his way back to God. In addition to prayer, the chaplain could have opened other resources that were available.

Background information that the practitioner considers useful:

Stephen B. Roberts, ed., *Professional Spiritual and Pastoral Care: A Practical Clergy and Chaplain's Handbook*. Woodstock, VT: SkyLight Paths, 2012.

Reality Testing and Meditation for a New Widow

Description of the client's circumstances and the spiritual care offered:

Late one evening the chaplain attended the death of a 28-year-old male who had died from an alcohol/drug overdose. His 21-year-old wife responded with near-fainting spells and was surrounded by more than 30 family members who were also openly grieving. Early the next day the wife returned to the hospital, asking the valet at the hospital door how to get a death certificate. She proceeded to tell the valet that she was fearful she might lose her children and her house. The valet came to the chaplaincy office and informed the chaplain of the distressed woman. The chaplain returned with the valet. The wife, appearing disheveled, sleep-deprived, and frightened, recognized the chaplain. Her hands were shaking and she displayed a flat affect. She expressed that she needed a death certificate to prove to child services that her husband was gone so they would not take her children away.

The chaplain suggested that they sit in a quiet room to talk for a few minutes. The wife declined, saying that someone was waiting for her in the car. The chaplain encouraged the wife to sit nearby, to which she agreed. The chaplain said, "Look at me.

Take a breath in and let it out. Can you do that a few times? Slowly . . ." The wife looked into the chaplain's eyes and *began breathing deeply*. The chaplain inquired if she had slept since last night. "I can't sleep. I haven't slept for three nights." The chaplain responded that this had been a time of suffering for her.

Again the wife asked about the death certificate. The chaplain explained what the coroner had told her the previous night, that there would not be a certificate until the autopsy was completed. There was not anything the wife needed to do until the funeral home called her. The chaplain stated that she cared about the wife and emphasized that the wife's job was to grieve and take care of herself. The wife stated that she would feel guilty for not taking care of her children. Her sister was watching them at the moment. The chaplain encouraged the woman to allow family to care for the children while she cared for herself. "But then everyone will think I am a terrible mother," she replied. The chaplain assured her that asking family to care for her children qualified her as a good mother. The chaplain encouraged her to sleep, cry, or take walks. These activities would help her be a better mother. The wife was concerned that she would never stop crying once she started. The chaplain remarked that tears come and go and are a part of normal grief. The chaplain shared how she herself would cry in the shower, which helped wash away the tears.

The wife *began to talk* about not having enough money for the funeral or the mortgage. "You are fearful of many things that will change with your husband gone. It is frightening to know he isn't here anymore," the chaplain responded. The wife spoke of how her husband used to reassure her, saying everything would be okay and that he loved her. Now she was worried about "going crazy" because she thought she had seen her late husband that morning. The chaplain stated that many people have visions of their late loved ones.

The chaplain had been learning the use of meditation with patients and asked if the wife would like to try an exercise to decrease worry. She *agreed*, and the chaplain led her in a 10-minute meditation, saying words such as "His love surrounds me" or

"He is here with me" (referring to the late husband). The wife's *breathing became more regular* as she did this, and afterward she *stated that she felt good*. The chaplain suggested other ways to minimize her worries, such as writing down actions needed and delegating tasks.

A phone call from a family member informed the wife that Medicaid would pay for the funeral, which gave her great relief. Then the wife started sharing her worry about the mortgage and food. When the chaplain suggested that life most likely had not been perfect with her husband, the wife *noted her fearfulness* when he would drink. The chaplain remarked that the wife had always taken responsibility for the family and was stronger than she realized, adding that her family could help her and that churches have grief support groups. The wife *affirmed these suggestions as possibilities*. The chaplain asked the wife if she would work on self-care that week, to which she replied that a friend would be coming to help sort pictures for a collage. Again the chaplain mentioned the need for the wife to sleep. She *said she would try*, and the chaplain, due at a meeting, said good-bye.

Description of what the practitioner, upon reflection, considers most appropriate:

The chaplain identified several things she could have done differently in this situation. First, it would have been helpful to either speak with the wife's driver or ask the valet to tell that person that the wife would return in about 20 minutes. This would have set time limits for the conversation, assured the wife that her driver was aware of the situation, and perhaps helped her relax enough to go to a quiet room for the conversation.

Second, when the wife mentioned that she thought she had seen her late husband, it may have been helpful to ask to hear more. This could have led to a life review or additional information about the wife's needs.

Third, the chaplain learned that it is not healthy to suggest that an individual meditate on another person's love. This promotes codependency, so it would be preferable to use a form of divine love or perhaps love from the higher self instead.

Lastly, even if the chaplain knows the protocol for obtaining a death certificate or dealing with child services, it is best to refer those questions to specialized staff. This allows the chaplain to focus on emotions and spiritual care.

Background information that the practitioner considers useful:

Joyce D. Davidson and Kenneth J. Doka, eds., *Living with Grief at Work, at School, at Worship*. Washington DC: Hospice Foundation of America, 1999. 5,7.

Kenneth J. Doka, ed., *Living with Grief after Sudden Loss*. Washington DC: Hospice Foundation of America, 1996. 11,145–146.

Jeanne Stevenson Moessner, ed., *Through the Eyes of Women: Insights for Pastoral Care*. Minneapolis: Augsburg Fortress, 1996. 304.

David K. Switzer, *Pastoral Care Emergencies: Ministering to People in Crisis*. Mahwah, NJ: Paulist Press, 1989. 45, 49.

Reality-Testing Hope in Terminal Illness

Description of the client's circumstances and the spiritual care offered:

This was the fourth or fifth visit the chaplain had made to a married 53-year-old patient with a diagnosis of recurrent ovarian cancer. She had been referred to him as a terminal patient.

In previous visits, they had talked about her medical condition—a history of several gynecological and intestinal tumors and a number of surgeries for them, in addition to the current surgery. Her cancer was found at a fairly late stage, and she did not have chemotherapy because of some misunderstandings between her and her previous doctor. She expressed trust in her new doctor, believing that he would be able to prescribe the right chemo mix to attack whatever cancer was left in her. She was very hopeful and trusting that God was going to heal her through chemotherapy. The chaplain did not want to quash her hope, but given what she had told him and what her chart and her nurse said, he wondered how realistic her hope was and how she would respond if she were not healed. He was hoping to be able to address that in this visit.

The visit began with some general greetings and introduction to the patient's husband, whom the chaplain had not met before. One of the first things he noticed was that the patient was coloring in a coloring book. She said it was because she felt bored and it was keeping her mind occupied. She said that she was looking forward to being able to get out of bed later that day and to going home in a day or two.

The chaplain asked, "What is helping you to get through this time of being confined to bed?" She replied that she simply kept her trust in God, and that God was getting her through day by day. After an empathetic response, the chaplain wondered, "What would it be like if the chemotherapy did not get all the cancer?" With anxiety she responded quickly with, "Oh no, I don't think negative thoughts. I just focus on the positive. God is going to heal me; I know he is!" After the chaplain's active listening response, she anxiously asked, "*Please pray for me* that God will heal me."

With her husband holding one of her hands and the chaplain holding the other, he prayed, "God, we pray for your daughter right now. Please do bring your healing touch to her. Guide the hands of the doctor and others involved in her care. Give her the strength and patience to get through this and help her faith to remain strong. Amen."

Description of what the practitioner, upon reflection,
considers most appropriate:

Later the chaplain decided that his question about the chemotherapy not being a success did not work well. Another way to proceed with someone who is (desperately) hoping a treatment will be a cure or will prolong life might be something like "It sounds like you might still have some things you want to do in your life. Can you tell me about some of those things?" After hearing about those things, one might ask, "What, if anything, can you be doing now to begin to accomplish some of those things?" Or, "I surely hope that the treatment does give you some more time to do those things. None of us really knows when we will die. I don't know when I will die. Can anything be done right now to work on getting those things done?" This kind of response would have focused more on the present moment and on the hope of being able to do more things in this life.

Background information that the practitioner considers useful:

Elisabeth Kübler-Ross, *On Death and Dying*. London: Macmillan, 1969.

Resistance in Anticipatory Grief

Description of the client's circumstances
and the spiritual care offered:

While making rounds in the ICU, the chaplain was approached by a nurse who indicated that a family was having difficulty making end-of-life care decisions for an elderly male patient. The chaplain was introduced to the patient's daughter-in-law. Her husband, the patient's only child, was away on military service. The daughter-in-law glanced at the chaplain but then avoided all eye contact. The room was dimly lit and a religious program was on the TV. The patient was wearing an oxygen mask and moved restlessly in his restraint. His eyes were open and unfocused. He would occasionally try to talk, but his speech was slurred and incoherent.

After introducing herself to the daughter-in-law, the chaplain indicated her awareness of the seriousness of the situation and asked if she could be of assistance to both the patient and to her. The daughter-in-law said that she did not want anything. The chaplain's empathetic comment about the difficulty in reaching the husband was rebuffed, and eye contact continued to be avoided. The daughter-in-law stated dismissively that both she and her father-in-law were Christians and then stepped out of the room, cell phone in hand. The chaplain met with a similar reaction later in the evening.

A week later, the chaplain found the patient, his son, daughter-in-law, and grandson in another unit. She established rapport with the son, but the daughter-in-law again avoided eye contact and left shortly with the grandson to get something to eat. When the chaplain asked the husband whether they would prefer a male chaplain, the son said that would not be necessary. He *gladly accepted* the chaplain's offer of prayer and thereafter said he would tell his wife that she was remembered in that prayer.

Description of what the practitioner, upon reflection, considers most appropriate:

If the chaplain had acknowledged the daughter-in-law's obvious concern for the patient at the outset, thereby validating her feelings and providing an opportunity for her to express her grief, the resistance might have been lessened. At the same time the chaplain could have been more inwardly at peace with making a graceful exit if she perceived that the daughter-in-law simply was not open to receiving her care. Also, in the later visit with the son, given the rapport she had established with him, the chaplain could have gently followed up on the nurse's concern about end-of-life-care decision making.

Background information that the practitioner considers useful:

Richard Dana, Lewis Bernstein, and Rosalyn S. Bernstein, *Interviewing: A Guide for Health Professionals.* New York: Appleton-Century Crofts, 1985.

Glendon Moriarty, *Pastoral Care of Depression: Helping Clients Heal Their Relationship with God.* New York: Haworth, 2006.

Sailor Feeling Helpless, Angry, and Trapped

Description of the client's circumstances and the spiritual care offered:

A 22-year-old sailor on duty overseas sought counsel from the chaplain. He was the father of a two-month-old child with birth defects: a heart defect and a few organs not in the right place. The family lived in the United States where the child could receive care—corrective surgeries—and be nurtured by the sailor's young wife.

The sailor *shared* with the chaplain his feelings of helplessness as a father and husband away from his family; his anger with life and God for his child being born this way; his feeling trapped by the job and life; his tiredness in being on edge and having to grow up quickly. The weight of the situation was depressing him and weighing him down.

The chaplain "simply listened. He needed a 'safe' place to let go." As the sailor talked, he cried a few times. As he spoke, in appropriate places, the chaplain repeated back what the younger man said to him so he knew the chaplain was listening. The chaplain also asked a few questions along the way to move him to come up with his own options and resolution for the situation, both in the short-term and long-term.

The sailor believed in God, so they "tapped into the spiritual resources he needed as well as tangible ones." With the sailor's permission, the chaplain prayed to end the session and then set a follow-up appointment.

Description of what the practitioner, upon reflection, considers most appropriate:

In retrospect the chaplain "would have done it the same way again. For this situation it was effective." After their initial meeting, the young man continued "to be proactive in enjoying himself with his resources to intentionally build his faith to move him and his family through this tough time."

Sense of Hopelessness after Terminal Diagnosis

Description of the client's circumstances
and the spiritual care offered:

The chaplain visited a 35-year-old female after she had been told that her cancer of the brain was inoperable. She *shared her anger and desperation*, for she felt that her life was just beginning. The chaplain listened carefully and asked questions to help explore her feelings. He wanted to help her process the information about her diagnosis and what it meant for her emotionally, relationally, and physically. She *asked the chaplain to visit again* as she *reached out for him to hold her hand*, giving him a sense that his supportive and comforting efforts were appreciated.

Description of what the practitioner, upon reflection,
considers most appropriate:

If given the opportunity to repeat the encounter, the chaplain would reflect more deeply on the meaning of the patient's body language and review her chart in advance to obtain more information. Further, he would also check in with a trusted colleague regarding countertransference implications. In other words, was there a "ghost" in the room—someone from the chaplain's own life whom he was projecting onto the patient and her experience?

Background information that the practitioner considers useful:

Wayne E. Oates, *The Minister's Own Mental Health*. New York: Channel, 1961.

Separation, Isolation, and Worry
in Ill Infant's Mother

Description of the client's circumstances
and the spiritual care offered:

On initial assessment rounds in the pediatrics unit, the chaplain found a one-year-old girl in respiratory distress, a serious condition for very young children and typically treated aggressively by the medical team. The chaplain also knew that the patient would not be alone but would most likely be with at least one parent. The chaplain did not know if this was a first child or the age of the parent. Her experience informed her that young mothers (late teens to early twenties) are ill-prepared to deal with health crises with their babies. Not only are the babies distressed, but often the mother is unable to cope emotionally with the situation. The chaplain went into the encounter with the expectation that she might be providing some mentoring for such an ill-prepared young mother, along with any emotional and spiritual support that she usually offered.

When the mother returned to the crib, she was wary, but she *relaxed* upon seeing the chaplain's name badge, being introduced, and picking up on the chaplain's intentionally relaxed manner. The mother *quickly dove into her story*, saying that she and her husband had moved a great distance from her own family and culture into the immediate area only the previous week, as he had found a job near his parents' home. She even shared her concern that she might be pregnant again. An excerpt of their conversation follows:

Mother: "I'd never been away from home. Lived there all my life. This place is different. I don't have my mom and dad or my sisters here. Just (Husband)'s folks."

Chaplain: "You don't have the mountains here or family. I'd guess you're a bit homesick."

Mother: (cries quietly) "Yeah. We move here, and right away (Baby) and I are in a hospital. And I can't help my baby."

Then a bit later:

Chaplain: "(Mother), may I pray with you? Would that help?"
Mother: "Sure. (Baby) and I need a prayer."

The chaplain then prayed: "Lord of heaven and earth, we lift our eyes to the hills from whence comes our help. Our help is you, O Lord. You watch over us day and night, tenderly like a mother, giving us what we need each day, filling us with hope. Be with (Baby) and (Mother) this evening. Bring healing to little (Baby)'s body so that she can leave here. Bring peace of mind and heart to (Mother) as she learns to live in a new place. Let her know that you are with her every step of the way. Heavenly Father, we trust you and hope in you. Thank you for giving us Jesus, in whose name we pray. Amen." The mother *thanked* the chaplain, who said she'd have a chaplain check by in the morning. Then the chaplain took her leave with a blessing, "Peace be with you."

Description of what the practitioner, upon reflection, considers most appropriate:

In retrospect the chaplain felt that she may have "overidentified with the patient's mother and made assumptions" about what the mother might have felt "as a dislocated woman from Appalachia." A better response, according to the chaplain, would have been to "check in with her" to learn what exactly the mother found so "different for her in this new location." Regarding her spiritual care for the mother, the chaplain felt she needed "to slow down to find out [the mother's] religious background and what she felt she needed spiritually."

After the mother commented, "I don't have my mom and dad or my sisters here. Just (Husband's) folks," the chaplain would rather have said more simply, "I'd guess you're a bit homesick. What do you see as different here?" Also, instead of "May I pray with you?" she would rather have said, "(Mother), is there anything else I can do for you as a chaplain? What is your faith background?"

Background information that the practitioner considers useful:

Stephen B. Roberts, ed., *Professional Spiritual and Pastoral Care: A Practical Clergy and Chaplain's Handbook.* Woodstock, VT: SkyLight Paths, 2012.

Alfred L. Cooke, Michael Brazzel, and Argentine Saunders Craig, eds., *Reading Book for Human Relations Training,* 8th ed. Leesburg, VA: National Institute for Applied Behavioral Science (National Training Laboratory), 1999.

Shock at News of the Murder of a Loved One

Description of the client's circumstances
and the spiritual care offered:

The hospital chaplain on call met the arriving mother of a young adult male penal institution inmate who had been pronounced dead upon arrival at the ER. (The deceased had suffered violent injuries during incarceration at the hands of another inmate.) The mother, who appeared to be in her forties, was accompanied by two adult males in their twenties. They were as yet unaware of his death, but as the chaplain and family were meeting in the hallway, the mother "read" the chaplain's face and collapsed onto the floor in anguished wails. The chaplain enlisted the two men's help in assisting her to a small family room, where creature comforts were provided and the chaplain offered a prayer.

The chaplain acted as a go-between from the mother to staff and back, informing staff of her arrival and getting the doctor to check in with her. Later when the mother asked if she could see the body, the chaplain took her request to the staff, and relayed the word from the doctor that this could not be done because of the required murder investigation procedures that would take some time. He also conveyed the doctor's advice to return home and stand by for further guidance on how to proceed.

Throughout the process, the chaplain stayed close to the mother and repeatedly expressed his sadness and regret at this horrific event and its impact. As they were leaving, he accompanied the mother and one young man to the exit. When the other young man drove up in their car, the chaplain assisted her in getting seated. As she was settling in, she looked up and *expressed her thanks* to the chaplain.

Description of what the practitioner, upon reflection, considers most appropriate:

In a similar situation, the chaplain would make a greater effort to (1) not get caught up in the flood of emotion, (2) be careful to introduce himself and his role, (3) learn the names of all three people and their relationships to each other, and (4) use their names in prayers if prayers were wanted, with guidance from them regarding prayer content.

The chaplain would also elicit the family's religious preference and the deceased's story, and would strongly negotiate with staff regarding viewing to allow grieving and prayer if desired. He would also suggest involving a pastor of their choice, encouraging them to stay longer if desired, and providing a list of important contact numbers so that they could monitor the situation from home and know what they could do next.

Background Information that the practitioner considers useful:

George C. Kandle and Henry H. Cassler, *Ministering to Prisoners and Their Families*. New York: Prentice-Hall, 1968.

Sudden, Devastating Loss of a Child

Description of the client's circumstances and the spiritual care offered:

A child was rushed to the Emergency Department with breathing difficulty. A Code Blue (a hospital code used to indicate a patient requiring immediate resuscitation) was called for the child. The medical staff sprang into action and worked as a team feverishly to save the child, but the child died. The family went to pieces. It was a totally unexpected death.

The chaplain spent time with the staff and the family, offering support to them. He put his "arms around them, and they cried." He cried with them.

It was a terrible event, but both family and staff *acknowledged the helpfulness* of the chaplain's presence and support.

Description of what the practitioner, upon reflection, considers most appropriate:

In retrospect the chaplain wrote, "The best spiritual care in this case was to not say too much. I allowed the family to grieve in their own way. I told staff and other family members that [was okay] as long as they are not doing harm to themselves or anyone else."

The chaplain further reflected, "What I would have done differently was to involve more people (family members) in the pastoral care," encouraging family members to help one another.

Background information that the practitioner considers useful:

Judith Lewis Herman, *Trauma and Recovery: The Aftermath of Violence—from Domestic Abuse to Political Terror.* New York: Basic Books, 1992.

Terminal Patient of Faith, Hope-Filled until Death

Description of the client's circumstances and the spiritual care offered:

The chaplain was called to the ER for a 49-year-old married woman of faith and mother of two (a 23-year-old son and a 19-year-old daughter) who was being admitted. The patient was a breast cancer survivor, but she was now ill. Her spouse was with her. She underwent testing and scans; the results showed cancer in the brain, with a prognosis of three to four months of survival. The patient stated that she would fight and beat the disease with the help of God. The family was involved with a church.

The patient had several admissions, during which the chaplain was always present. Early in the relationship the chaplain conducted a brief ceremony in which she blessed the hands of the patient and her husband. The patient exhibited a strong hope throughout treatment, expressing in words and manner her love for God and for her family and friends. She never expressed or seemed to show any anger. She accepted that "God knows best."

In her final admission, she went into a coma. Shortly thereafter, her spouse made the decision to remove life support, and *asked for the chaplain's presence*. In those last moments, the chaplain and family members prayed, talked, and said good-byes. The team removed life support, and the patient died peacefully in a few moments.

Description of what the practitioner, upon reflection, considers most appropriate:

The chaplain had stayed present with the patient throughout various admissions, including during the coma, reading to her and holding the hands she had blessed. In her ongoing ministry, the chaplain had become very close to this patient and felt the patient's death to be a major loss in her own life.

In retrospect the chaplain felt deeply thankful—in particular for the relationships she had been able to develop with the patient, her family, her friends, and staff members. She felt especially grateful that she had blessed the hands of the patient early on, in part a symbol of her loving care.

The chaplain's strong sense of gratitude was centered in the divine grace and strength she felt she had received, since at the outset she had wondered whether she would be spiritually strong enough to continue this ministry until the patient's death.

Background information that the practitioner considers useful:

Kathleen Tuite, "Blessing of Hands Ceremony." Caldwell, NJ: Caldwell University Nursing Department. Unpublished.

Unexpected Terminal Diagnosis

Description of the client's circumstances
and the spiritual care offered:

On his first admission to a hospital since birth, the 53-year-old single, unemployed male learned that he had stage IV cancer, and that he had six to eight weeks to live. No treatment options were offered.

The patient used the morning after receiving this news to reflect on his life and made decisions about his faith and his need for God in his circumstance. He had visited the church where a particular minister was pastor, so he asked that minister to come to see him in the hospital.

Upon the minister's arrival in the patient's room, the patient *related the events of the previous day* and acknowledged his need for support and encouragement. He asked for a Bible and for prayer on his behalf. The patient had some *trouble talking without breaking into tears.* The minister acknowledged his story, offered his support and prayer, and affirmed the patient's faith and desire to let God be with him in the coming days.

Description of what the practitioner, upon reflection,
considers most appropriate:

In retrospect the minister felt that there was not much he could offer other than a listening ear and an attentive posture. The patient had been traumatized by the news of his illness. His world had been dramatically altered. Restatement, reflection, and affirmation of God's care and grace were "all" the minister responded with. [*Editor's note:* "All" was "a lot."]

Background information that the practitioner considers useful:

G. Fackre, "Ministry of Presence," *Dictionary of Pastoral Care and Counseling.* Nashville: Abingdon, 1990. 950–951.

Harold S. Kushner, *When Bad Things Happen to Good People.* New York: Schocken, 1981.

Afterword

Henry G. Heffernan, SJ, staff chaplain with the National Institutes of Health, originated this collection by adapting a cognitive therapy training template for use in Clinical Pastoral Education (CPE). The project was introduced into CPE curricula and piloted with several intern groups and one resident group in the East Central ACPE Region during 2006–2008. Based on student and educator critiques, a revised protocol was developed. Early samples were later edited to conform to a standard format.

From 2008 to 2012, the Editor collected samples of pastoral care and spiritual care interventions, not only from students who had refined their accounts of patient visits in light of feedback from their CPE peers and supervisors, but also from workshop papers written by experienced chaplains, community clergy, and educators. In addition to the purposes cited in the Preface, this collection provides opportunities for replicable research toward the evidence-based pastoral/spiritual care best practices that are essential to ever-higher quality caregiving in congregations and to compliance with ever-higher standards in modern health care.

The Editor thanks the collection's innovator and first editor, Henry Heffernan; the several hundred students, practitioners, and educators who contributed papers; the ACPE Research Network coordinator, John Ehman, and Leigh McMillan Avery, for IT support; workshop leaders Ralph Ciampa, Yoke Lye Lim Kwong, Paul Steinke, and James Travis; and Connie Bonner and Yoke Lye Lim Kwong, CPE supervisors whose students provided the highest number of papers nationally.

Index